·tr

PRACTICAL
OPHTHALMIC LENSES

First published, 1974
Reprinted, 1979
Second edition, 1983
Reprinted, 1987
Third edition, 1990
Reprinted, 1996
Reprinted, 1997
Reprinted, 1999
Reprinted, 2002

© **Butterworth & Co (Publishers) Ltd, 1983**

British Library Cataloguing in Publication Data

Jalie, M.
    Practical ophthalmic lenses.—3rd ed.
    1. Lenses
    I. Title   II. Wray L.
    617.7'52   RE976

    ISBN 0 900099 25 9

This edition is printed by kind permission of
Butterworth Scientific Ltd., Guildford, Surrey, England.

Printed and bound in the UK by MPG Information Division, Unwin Brothers Limited,
The Gresham Press, Old Woking, Surrey, GU22 9LH.

Practical Ophthalmic Lenses

Third Edition

M. JALIE
SMSA, FBDO(Hons), Hon CGIA, MBIM
Head of Department of Applied Optics,
City and East London College, London

L. WRAY
BSc(Lond), FBCO, DOrth, DCLP, MBIM
Former Head of Department of Applied Optics,
City and East London College, London

Association of British Dispensing Opticians

PREFACE TO THE THIRD EDITION

A number of books on ophthalmic and dispensing optics have been published in recent years, but they tend to omit elementary practical instruction.

This book is based upon lectures given and practical work done in the Department of Applied Optics at the City and East London College, London, and includes several original experiments.

The experimental sequence has been planned to provide an integrated introduction to the applied optics of ophthalmic lenses. In general the experiments are deliberately designed so that equipment is kept to a minimum. This will assist the smaller optical firm or practice in formulating a training scheme. The more advanced experiments, those marked with an asterisk in the contents list, can be omitted at the first reading.

The original sequence of 72 experiments in the first edition has been unaltered. Experiments 73 − 88 give a system of surfacing instruction which to our knowledge does not exist elsewhere. It will enable the surfacing laboratory to obtain more accurate solutions to lens thickness problems which at present can be tackled only by approximate methods of trial and error. The concluding experiments reflect the comments we have received from professional staff in the ophthalmic optical industry that certain aspects of thick ophthalmic lenses and prisms should be given more detailed treatment.

Examples of simple computer programs are given.

Appendices are provided at the end of the book which will allow the student's or trainee's progress to be assessed periodically. A suggested marking scheme for these tests is included.

We hope that the book will have a wide application. It will be found useful by opticians, optometrists, optical technicians, manufacturing firms and optical receptionists, and for teaching purposes. The book complements existing ophthalmic textbooks.

The authors would be pleased to receive any comments which could be used to improve the contents or widen the usefulness of the book.

M. J.
L. W.

CONTENTS

CONTENTS

*These more advanced experiments can be omitted at the first reading (*see* Preface).

CONTENTS

*These more advanced experiments can be omitted at the first reading (*see* Preface).

CONTENTS

*These more advanced experiments can be omitted at the first reading (*see* Preface).

CONTENTS

APPENDICES

Experiment 1
OPTICAL ELEMENTS

Theory

This experiment is an introduction to some of the various types of lenses and prisms. The term 'optical element' can be used for any transparent material which has been optically worked.

All optical elements have some effect on light incident upon them. Light may be reflected by a mirror, be transmitted by a glass block or lens, be partially absorbed (or reflected) by a tinted lens, or suffer a change in direction by a prism. If you look through a plus lens at a near object, the object is seen magnified. This is not so with a minus lens, where the object is diminished in size.

Apparatus

Box containing numbered set of optical elements; target consisting of two perpendicular black lines on white card.

Procedure

(1) Note the number of the optical element.

(2) Handle it with your fingers and note whether it is a plus or minus lens or a prism. If the optical element has plane surfaces inclined to each other, it is a prism. Note whether the element is glass or plastics.

(3) If it is a lens, look through it at a *near* object. Is the object seen magnified? If so, it is a plus lens.

(4) Hold the optical element approximately 8–10 cm from the eye and view through it the crossline target distant 4-6 metres. Move the optical element

      (a) laterally

      (b) by rotation

and note what happens.

(5)   Place the optical element on a sheet of white paper to observe whether it is tinted.

(6)   Record any other observations you wish to make.

(7)   Imagine that the optical element has been cut down the middle; draw what you think would be the cross-sectional appearance of the optical element.

Record your results under the headings shown below.

Optical element No.	Material	Lens		Prism	Tint	Optical element	
		Plus	Minus			Moved laterally	Rotated

Experiment 2
LAWS OF REFLECTION

Theory

With the aid of the ray box we can trace the path of light at incidence and reflection from a mirror and hence verify the laws of reflection.

Apparatus

Drawing board, plane mirror, ray box, ruler, protractor.

Procedure

Draw a line BC on the paper to mark the position of the plane mirror *(Figure 2.1)*. Arrange the ray box so that only one ray DA emerges from it. Draw a perpendicular (to the mirror) AE on the paper. This is termed the normal to the mirror.

Ray DA is reflected at A to become ray AF. $<$ DAE is the angle of incidence i, EAF is the angle of reflection i'.

By rotating the ray box, keeping the ray incident at the point A, various values of i and corresponding values of i' can be measured with the protractor. Take at least six readings and tabulate your results as follows, and plot a graph of i against i'.

Angle of incidence i	Angle of reflection i'

Exercises

(1) What is the slope of the graph? Show that the value of the slope verifies the law of reflection that the angle of incidence equals the angle of reflection. (*Answer:* slope of graph is unity.)

(2) A ray of light is incident on a plane mirror and the angle formed between the incident and the reflected beam is 60°. What is the angle between the reflected beam and the mirror. (*Answer:* 60°.)

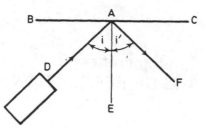

*Figure 2.1. BC represents the plane
mirror, A is the point of incidence of
the ray of light emitted by the ray
box, AE is the normal to the mirror
surface. The ray DA is reflected by
the mirror, the reflected ray being
AF. Measure the angle of incidence i
and the angle of reflection i'. Note
that angles i and i'are measured from
the rays to the normal*

(3)   If the angle between an incident beam and a plane mirror is
35°, what are the angles of incidence and reflection. (*Answer:* 55°.)

(4)   The angle of incidence at a plane mirror is 40°. What deviation
will the light suffer by reflection? (*Answer:* 100°.)

Check the above examples by (a) calculation and (b) use of the ray
box and the protractor.

Experiment 3
NEUTRALIZATION OF SPHERICAL
LENSES

Theory

The measurement of the focal power of lenses can be done in many ways. Two main methods are used for ophthalmic lenses:
(1) Neutralization.
(2) Vertex power measuring instruments.
This experiment is restricted to neutralization of spherical lenses.

In *Figure 3.1*, ABDC represents the cross section of a rectangular glass block. Ray QO is incident normally to the plane faces AOC, BGD and emerges undeviated from the block. Let us assume that this glass block is made into a lens whose cross section is represented by EOFG.

For a very narrow region around the points O and G the lens is in effect a rectangular piece of glass, hence the incident ray QO is still undeviated after passing through the lens. Any other incident ray XY parallel to QO will be deviated after passing through the lens. Ray QO is said to pass through the optical centre of the lens, which is commonly regarded as coinciding with the vertex of either surface when the lens is considered thin.

Figure 3.2a shows a thin spherical lens of positive focal power. An incident ray BO passes through the optical centre O of the lens and is undeviated. A transverse movement of the lens is made so that the incident ray passing through the point B parallel to the optical axis is refracted in the direction CD. An observer looking along CD appears to see a movement of the image of B from the position B to the position B'. From *Figure 3.2b* it can be seen that the movement of the lens and the movement of the image are in opposite directions. This is termed an 'against' movement. It is an indication that the lens has positive focal power: the more powerful the lens, the greater the apparent movement of the object seen through the lens for a given transverse movement of the lens.

Figure 3.3a and *b* shows a thin spherical lens of negative focal power. The lens is moved as indicated in the diagram and there is an apparent transverse movement of the object seen through the lens in the same direction as that in which the lens is moved; the image of the

Figure 3.1. *ABDC is a rectangular block of glass. Ray QO is incident normally upon the face AC and emerges without deviation from face BD at the point G. The faces AC and BD are now surfaced to produce the biconvex lens EOFG. For the narrow region OG, the lens can be considered to remain a parallel block of glass and ray QO is still undeviated. Ray XY, however, is refracted by the lens and emerges at the point Z from the surface EGF*

(a)   (b)

Figure 3.2. *'Against' movement produced by plus lens under the transverse test*

object point B has moved from B to B' and an eye looking through the lens views the image along CD. This is termed a 'with' movement. It is an indication that the lens has negative focal power. Hence by the observation of 'against' or 'with' movements one can make an estimation of the focal power of a lens. This is called the transverse test.

6

NEUTRALIZATION OF SPHERICAL LENSES

The focal power of a thin spectacle lens can be determined by placing lenses of opposite sign in contact with the spectacle lens until no movement is discernible with the transverse test; this is called neutralization.

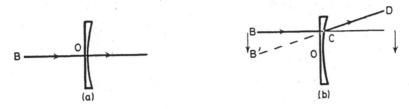

Figure 3.3. 'With' movement produced by minus lens under the transverse test

Apparatus

Box of spherical lenses of unknown focal power; neutralizing set or trial case; crossline chart.

Procedure

(1) If the lenses are numbered, arrange the lenses in numerical order and record your results as 4.1, 4.2 . . . which would indicate the first and second lens of box No. 4.

(2) Take the first lens, hold it before the eye and apply the transverse test, viewing the crossline chart through the lens.

(3) Make a rough estimation of the focal power and record the sign of the unknown lens. If this lens gives a with movement, record a minus sign.

(4) If the estimation is −1.50 D, take from the trial case a lens of focal power +1.50 D. Place the two lenses in contact; avoid scratching or damaging the lens surfaces. Apply again the transverse test.

(5) If a with movement is observed, select another neutralizing lens of greater focal power. Apply the transverse test. Repeat, increasing the focal power of the neutralizing lens in systematic steps until the transverse test shows an against movement.

(6) An against movement indicates that the power of the neutralizing lens is greater than that of the unknown lens. Reduce the power of the neutralizing lens for the next observation. Repeat if necessary until the transverse test shows no movement. The unknown lens is then neutralized; record this result.

7

(7) Record also:

(a) The focal power and sign of the neutralizing lens which just gives an against movement.

(b) The focal power and sign of the neutralizing lens which just gives a with movement.

(8) It may be necessary for unknown lenses of high focal power to be neutralized by a combination of two neutralizing lenses.

Experiment 4
REFLECTION FROM A ROTATING
MIRROR

Theory

This is a continuation of Experiment 2, and is to verify that if the direction of an incident ray on a plane mirror is constant, a rotation of the mirror through angle θ will cause a rotation of the reflected ray through angle 2θ.

Apparatus

As for Experiment 2.

Procedure

Arrange the experimental set-up as in *Figure 2.1*.

Rotate the mirror BAC in an anti-clockwise direction through angle θ, keeping the position of the ray box and hence the direction of the incident ray DA unchanged.

The reflected ray will now lie not along the direction AF but along a new direction between AC and AF. Measure the rotation of the reflected ray α and the angle of rotation of the mirror θ.

Repeat the experiment for at least three values of θ.

Tabulate your results as follows.

θ	α	2θ

Plot a graph of α against θ.

Exercises

(1) If the mirror is silvered on the back surface, the lines representing the incident and reflected rays may not meet on the mirror surface.

Give reasons for this. (Hint: incident ray is refracted at the first surface.)

(2) What does the value of the slope of the graph indicate?

(3) Give a geometrical proof of the result of this experiment.

(4) Give an example of an instrument using a rotating mirror.

(5) A source of light and a screen are in the same plane. A mirror is parallel with the screen and distant 2 metres from it and a patch of light is reflected on the screen. How far will the patch move when the mirror is rotated 4°? (*Answer:* 28.1 cm.)

Experiment 5
THE SURFACE POWER AND FORM OF
SPHERICAL OPHTHALMIC LENSES

Theory

The surfaces of the biconvex lens in *Figure 5.1* are portions of the spheres having centres at C_1 and C_2. The line $C_1 C_2$ is the optical axis and intersects the lens at O, the optical centre. If the surfaces each have the same radius, then the lens is termed equiconvex. *Figure 5.2* shows sections of the various forms of spherical ophthalmic lenses.

The figures denote the surface power in dioptres of each lens. The sum of the surface powers gives the focal power of the lens *if it is thin*, and in the two examples shown is +4.00 D and −4.00 D respectively.

The front surface of a spectacle lens is always the more convex or less concave; in *Figure 5.2* the front surface of each lens is to the left.

This experiment is a further example of neutralization and will enable you to determine the 'form' of the spectacle lens.

Apparatus

Neutralizing set, crossline chart, marking ink and pen, straight edge (ruler), lens measure, assorted spherical lenses.

Procedure

When a lens is being neutralized, the neutralizing lens should be actually in contact with the *back* surface of the lens being tested. This cannot of course be done with a meniscus lens as *Figure 5.3* shows, hence the neutralizing lens is placed in contact with the front surface of the lens being tested. If the meniscus lens is thick and of high positive power, errors are introduced by this method. A later experiment will deal with this problem and it is ignored here.

11

(1)   Apply the transverse test and sort the lenses into positive and negative groups.

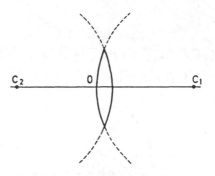

Figure 5.1. C_1 is the centre of curvature of the first surface. C_2 is the centre of curvature of the second surface. The line joining C_1 and C_2 is the optical axis of the lens. O is the optical centre of the lens – the lens being assumed to be infinitely thin

(a)

(b)

Figure 5.2. Forms of ophthalmic lenses. (a) Four forms in which a + 4.00 D lens might be made. (b) Four forms in which a − 4.00 D lens might be made

(2)   Mark the optical centre of each lens. This is the intersection of the crosslines seen through the lens as indicated in *Figure 5.4. Figures 5.4a* and *b* represent the appearances through a positive and negative lens respectively.

(3)   Determine the focal power of each lens by neutralization and record this.

(4)   Test your ruler to check that it is a true straight edge. Place it carefully in contact with the surface of the lens so that it passes

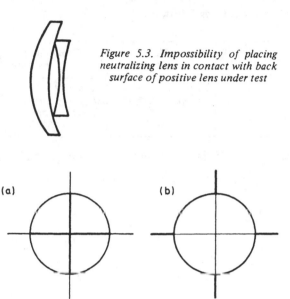

Figure 5.3. Impossibility of placing neutralizing lens in contact with back surface of positive lens under test

(a)   (b)

Figure 5.4. Appearance of crossline chart viewed through centred (a) positive lens and (b) negative lens

through the optical centre. Record the power of the surface as convex or positive if the ruler is in contact only at the centre, and concave or negative if in contact at the edge. If the lens is plano, the ruler will be in contact throughout its length. For shallow curves the edge and lens should be viewed against a well illuminated background. Repeat the procedure for the second surface of the lens.

(5)   Repeat step (4) without the straight edge, using only your thumb and forefinger to determine the form of the lens. This is to give you experience in the 'feel' of lenses of various powers. Do not record any results.

(6)   After steps (1) to (5) have been recorded, the lens measure is used to record the surface powers of the lens. Check the accuracy of the lens measure and allow for zero error. Hold the lens measure between the thumb and forefinger and place a third finger in contact

with the lens surface. Slowly lower the lens measure on to the lens surface, sliding it against the third finger. Make sure that the lens measure is perpendicular to the lens surface. Record the surface powers F_1 and F_2 of the lens.

Record your results as follows.

Lens No.	Focal power by neutralization	Form of lens using straight edge		Form of lens using lens measure		
		Front surface	Back surface	Front surface power F_1	Back surface power F_2	Focal power $F_1 + F_2$

Compare the results obtained by the lens measure and by neutralization.

Experiment 6
REFLECTION OF LIGHT AT TWO MIRRORS IN SUCCESSION

Theory

When light is reflected at two plane mirrors in succession, the deviation of the incident ray is twice the exterior angle between the mirrors and is therefore independent of the angle of incidence at the first mirror.

In *Figure 6.1*, plane mirrors M_1 and M_2 are inclined at angle a. An incident ray AB is reflected at mirror M_1 and is deviated in direction through angle d_1 along BC. At M_2 ray BC is reflected and the final direction of the incident ray AB after two reflections is along CD. Hence the total deviation of the incident ray AB is d_1 and d_2.

Let AB make an angle of incidence i_1 with mirror M_1.
Let BC make an angle of incidence i_2 with mirror M_2.

From the diagram *(Figure 6.1)*,
$$d_1 = 180 - 2i_1$$
$$d_2 = 180 - 2i_2$$
$$d_1 + d_2 = 360 - 2(i_1 + i_2) \ldots (1)$$

In triangle EBC,
$$\angle EBC = 90 - i_1$$
$$\angle ECB = 90 - i_2$$
$$\angle EBC + \angle ECB = 180 - (i_1 + i_2) \qquad \ldots (2)$$

But $\angle EBC + \angle ECB = 180 - a$ $\qquad \ldots (3)$

$\therefore$ from equations (2) and (3), $a = i_1 + i_2$,
and substituting this value in equation (1),
$$d_1 + d_2 = 360 - 2a$$
$$= 2(180 - a),$$ which is twice the exterior angle between the mirrors.

In optical instruments, mirrors are sometimes replaced by reflecting prisms.

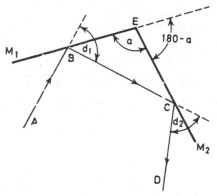

Figure 6.1. Two mirrors M_1 and M_2 are inclined at an angle a. Ray AB is reflected in the direction BC and is deviated by the first mirror through an angle d_1. At the second mirror, ray BC is deviated through an angle d_2 into the final direction CD. The total deviation of the incident ray AB after one reflection at each mirror is $d_1 + d_2$

Apparatus

Drawing board, two plane mirrors, ray box, pins, protractor.

Procedure

(1)   Place the two mirrors vertically on the paper inclined to each other at an angle of approximately $120°$. Arrange the ray box so that only one ray is emergent from it and that this undergoes reflection at each mirror. Draw the path of the ray ABCD. Measure the angle between the mirrors and the deviations d_1 and d_2.

Replace the mirrors but rotate both of them through $10°$ so that the angle a between the mirrors is unchanged. Arrange the ray box so that the direction of the reflected ray is parallel to that in the previous observation. Measure again the deviations d_1 and d_2.

Repeat the whole procedure with the mirrors inclined at an angle of $45°$. Record your results as follows, and give your conclusion.

a	2(180 − a)	d_1	d_2	$d_1 + d_2$

(2)   Place the two mirrors vertically on the paper inclined to each

other at an angle of $90°$. Place a pin between the mirrors. Find the number and positions of the images of the pin that can be seen. Repeat with the two mirrors inclined at an angle of (a) $60°$ and (b) $45°$.

It can be shown that the total number of images is $2\left(\dfrac{180}{a}\right) - 1$ when a has the above values. Do your observations verify this?

Exercises

(1) Explain the principle of the kaleidoscope.

(2) (a) Give diagrams showing two ways in which a beam of light may be deviated through $90°$ by plane mirrors.

(b) Give a diagram showing how a beam of light may be deviated through $90°$ by a right-angled prism.

(3) A ray reflected at two inclined mirrors is deviated by $100°$. What is the angle between the mirrors? (*Answer:* $130°$).

Experiment 7
CYLINDRICAL LENSES: THE ROTATION TEST

Theory

Eyes which suffer from the defect of astigmatism require correcting lenses whose powers vary in different meridians. The type of variation required is that the lenses should have a minimum power along one meridian, gradually increasing to a maximum power along a second meridian which lies at right angles to the first. These meridians of minimum and maximum power are known as the *principal meridians* of the lens. The simplest form of astigmatic lens is the *cylindrical lens*, which has no power along its minimum meridian, the surface curvature along this meridian being plane. The power of a cylindrical lens lies at right angles to this minimum meridian, the surface curvature along this maximum meridian being circular *(Figure 7.1)*.

Figure 7.1 illustrates positive and negative cylindrical lenses whose minimum meridians lie in the vertical meridian. Along the vertical meridians of the lens (BC, AA' or ED) there is no curvature. These meridians are parallel to the axis of revolution of the cylinder from which the lenses may be assumed to have been taken, and this direction is called the *axis direction* of the lenses. Along BE (or CD) the curvature of the cylindrical surface is a maximum and is circular. The direction BE or CD is called the *power meridian* of the cylinder. Along intermediate meridians between AA' and BE the surface curvature is elliptical.

If the axis meridian of a cylindrical lens is held vertically before a crossline chart and the transverse test is applied in the vertical meridian, no apparent movement of the crosslines will be detected since there is no power in the vertical meridian. If the lens is moved horizontally along its power meridian, this will cause the crosslines to move with the direction of the lens if the cylinder is negative and against the direction of the lens if the cylinder is positive. Along the power meridian the cylinder produces the same effects as a sphere.

18

When a spherical lens is rotated about its optical axis before a crossline chart, there is no effect upon the crosslines since all meridians of the spherical lens have the same power. A cylindrical lens rotated about its centre point will, however, produce an apparent rotation of the crosslines, an effect known as *scissors movement*. This scissors movement is exhibited by all astigmatic lenses, although the extent of the movement depends upon the power of the cylindrical element and the position of the lens in relation to the crosslines and the eye.

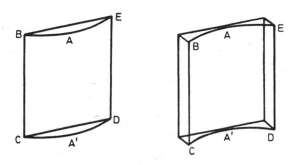

Figure 7.1. Plano-convex and plano-concave cylindrical lenses. BAEDA'C represents the cylindrical surface

When a cylindrical lens is rotated into such a position that its principal meridians, i.e., its axis and power meridians, are parallel to the limbs of the crossline chart, the limbs will appear unbroken as shown in *Figure 7.2*. This diagram shows the appearances obtained when a cylinder is held before the chart with its axis AA' parallel to the vertical limb of the chart.

Suppose that the cylinder of *Figure 7.2* is positive. When this lens is rotated in an anti-clockwise direction, say through 20°, the crosslines appear to 'scissor'; the vertical limb viewed through the lens rotates clockwise, in the opposite direction to the rotation of the lens *(Figure 7.3)*. This 'against' rotation of the vertical limb of the chart occurs whenever the limb is originally parallel to the axis meridian of a positive cylinder or the power meridian of a negative cylinder. The horizontal limb of the crosslines is seen in *Figure 7.3* to have rotated anti-clockwise, with the rotation of the lens. This 'with' rotation of the crossline limb occurs whenever the limb is originally parallel to the power meridian of a positive cylinder or the axis meridian of a negative cylinder.

If the cylinder shown in *Figure 7.2* is now supposed to be negative and the lens is rotated anti-clockwise, the appearance will be as shown

19

in *Figure 7.4*. The meridian AA' in *Figure 7.4* is the axis meridian of the negative cylinder and produces 'with' rotation as explained above. The horizontal crossline limb which was initially parallel to the power meridian of the negative cylinder is seen in *Figure 7.4* to have rotated against the direction of rotation of the lens.

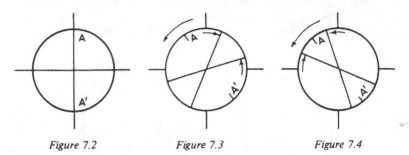

Figure 7.2   Figure 7.3   Figure 7.4

Figure 7.2. Scissors movement. View of crossline chart seen through astigmatic lens whose principal meridians are vertical and horizontal

Figure 7.3. If a positive cylinder axis vertical is rotated anti-clockwise, the vertical limb of the crossline chart seen through the lens rotates in an opposite direction and the horizontal limb of the chart seen through the lens rotates in the same direction

Figure 7.4. Appearance of the crosslines when a negative cylinder axis vertical is rotated anti-clockwise

By means of this rotation test we can at once differentiate between spherical and astigmatic lenses.

The meridian which produces against rotation is often called simply the 'plus axis' of an astigmatic lens. The 'plus axis' meridian is the axis meridian of a positive cylinder or the power meridian of a negative cylinder. The meridian which produces with rotation is called the 'minus axis' of an astigmatic lens. The 'minus axis' meridian is the axis meridian of a negative cylinder or the power meridian of a positive cylinder. It will be found in practice that it is easier to mark the position of the plus axis meridian of the lens than that of the minus axis, and the object of the following experiment is to mark the plus axis of a number of cylindrical or sphero-cylindrical lenses.

Apparatus

Box of astigmatic lenses; crossline chart (preferably in the form of a centration arm); fine pen and indian ink (or other marking implements).

Procedure

(1)   Hold the lens which is to be marked before the crossline chart, making sure that the extremities of the limbs may be viewed outside the lens periphery at the same time as the images of the lines seen through the lens. The back surface of the lens (if this is apparent) should be held nearer to the eye.

(2)   Rotate the lens until an unbroken appearance of the crosslines is obtained (as in *Figure 7.2*).

(3)   Make sure that the vertical meridian of the lens is the plus axis by a slight rotation, when the vertical limb rotates in the opposite direction, i.e., against the rotation of the lens.

(4)   Again obtain the unbroken appearance shown in *Figure 7.2* with the plus axis in the vertical meridian, and mark the extremities of the lens in this meridian with short lines as shown in *Figure 7.5*.

Figure 7.5. Two short vertical marks at the extremities of the lens show the axis direction of the cylinder

The direction indicated on the lens is the plus axis meridian of the lens and may be used to set the lens to an individual prescription (*see* Experiment 23).

Experiment 8
REFRACTIVE INDEX OF A GLASS OR PERSPEX BLOCK

Theory

Figure 8.1 shows a rectangular glass or Perspex block ABCD. Ray EF is incident at the point F and on passing into the glass block is changed in direction or refracted as FG. At G it undergoes another refraction and emerges as ray GH.

EF is the incident ray, AB is a boundary separating two optical media (in this case air and glass), and FG is the refracted ray.

The behaviour of light when it enters a new medium is governed by the laws of refraction, which are as follows.

(1) The incident ray EF, the normal to the surface at the point of incidence JF and the refracted ray FG all lie in one plane *(Figure 8.1)*.

(2) The ratio $\dfrac{\sin i}{\sin i'}$ is a constant for the glass and is called the refractive index. It is given the symbol n.

This experiment is to determine the refractive index of the block.

Apparatus

Ray box, drawing board, rectangular Perspex or glass block, protractor.

Procedure

(1) Set up the ray box to yield a single ray EF incident on the glass block ABCD as shown in *Figure 8.1*. Draw EF and the boundary of the glass block. Mark the point G where the ray FG emerges from the glass block. Remove the glass block and draw FG. Measure angles i and i'. Repeat for at least six values of i. Keep i values above 30° so that i

22

and i' can be measured with some accuracy. Plot a graph of sin i as ordinate against sin i' as abscissa. The value of the slope of the graph will be the refractive index of the glass.

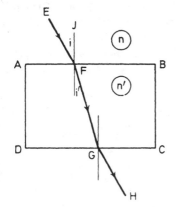

Figure 8.1. Ray EF makes an angle of incidence i with normal JF of the surface AB of the rectangular glass or Perspex block ABCD. The refracted ray makes an angle of refraction i' with the normal. A further refraction takes place at the other face of the block, and the emergent ray GH is parallel to the incident ray EF but laterally displaced

Record your result as follows.

i	sin i	i'	sin i'

(2)   This experiment is to demonstrate total internal reflection.

Set up the glass or Perspex as before. NM represents the single incident ray from the ray box making angle i with the normal LM on the short face of the rectangular glass block. Make i about 45° and position the point M of incident ray MN so that the refracted ray MO is incident at O on the face DC of the glass block. It will be found that the incident ray MO is not refracted from the glass block into the air but is totally internally reflected along OP according to the laws of reflection *(Figure 8.2)*.

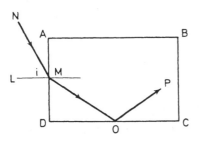

Figure 8.2. Ray MO, incident at O, is not refracted into air but is totally internally reflected inside the block, surface DC acting like a plane mirror

23

Exercises

(1) A ray of light is incident on a glass block at an angle of 52° with the normal. The angle of refraction is 31°. Calculate the refractive index of the glass block. (*Answer:* 1.53.)

(2) Note that the incident and emergent rays EF and GH are parallel to each other but laterally displaced. Explain why this is so.

(3) A beam of light is incident on a rectangular block of glass at an angle of incidence of 45° The refractive index of the glass block is 1.5. Trace the path of light through the glass block. (*Answer:* i' = 28°8'.)

Experiment 9
DETERMINATION OF THE CYLINDRICAL SURFACE AND AXIS DIRECTION BY THE STRAIGHT-EDGE TEST

Theory

In Experiment 5 the straight-edge test was applied to spherical lenses in order to determine the form of their surfaces. In this experiment we will extend this test to determine the form and axis direction of a cylindrical surface.

When a straight edge is rotated over a spherical surface, the amount of light which is seen beneath the edge remains the same.

Figure 9.1 shows a convex and a concave cylindrical surface. When a straight edge is applied to a cylindrical surface, the appearance depends upon the position of the edge in relation to the cylinder axis. If the straight edge is placed along the axis, the appearance will be exactly the same as if it had been placed upon a plane surface. No light will be seen beneath the edge. If the straight edge is placed along any other meridian it will be in contact only at the centre if the surface is convex, or at the edges if the surface is concave. Rotation of the straight edge along these intermediate directions will cause more, or less, light to be seen beneath the edge. By rotating a straight edge over a lens surface we can therefore determine whether the surface is cylindrical and also the approximate axis direction.

Apparatus

Box of flat astigmatic lenses; straight edge (e.g., a good metal ruler); crossline chart.

Procedure

(1)   Apply the rotation test, using the crossline chart, to verify that the lens is astigmatic.

(2)   Place the straight edge carefully in contact with the lens surface and hold up the lens before a distant light source. If light can be seen escaping beneath the edge, the surface is curved. The straight edge

Figure 9.1. Convex and concave cylindrical surfaces

may be on the spherical surface of the lens or along the power meridian or other intermediate meridian of a cylindrical surface. If no light can be seen beneath the edge, it may be in contact with a plane surface or it may be along the axis meridian of a cylindrical surface.

(3)   Rotate the lens beneath the straight edge. If the appearance remains the same, the surface is spherical or plane. If the amount of light seen beneath the edge increases or decreases, the surface is cylindrical.

(4)   When the cylindrical surface has thus been determined, the lens should be rotated beneath the straight edge until no light escapes between the edge and the surface. The meridian along which the straight edge lies is the axis meridian.

(5)   With this meridian held between finger and thumb, the lens may now be held up before the crossline chart and the axis direction marked correctly by the more sensitive appearance of continuous crosslines.

If the axis marking is performed on the cylindrical surface, it will enable you to identify this surface.

Experiment 10
DETERMINATION OF THE CYLINDRICAL SURFACE AND AXIS DIRECTION BY THE REFLECTION TEST

Theory

In the preceding experiment, the cylindrical surface and axis direction of an astigmatic lens were found by means of the straight-edge test. In this experiment we will consider an alternative method of performing this operation. The form of a surface may be determined by examining the images produced by reflection at the surface.

A plane surface produces an undistorted image of an object, whereas a curved surface produces a distorted image. A convex surface produces a diminished image (rather like a curved rear-view car mirror), whereas a concave surface produces an enlarged image (similar to that produced by a shaving mirror). These images can be examined by holding the lens up close to the eye, under the lower lid, and looking down on to the lens surface. The form of the surface determines the appearance of images of objects seen by reflection at the lens surface.

When the lens is rotated beneath the lower lid, the images produced by a spherical surface will remain unchanged, but if the surface is cylindrical the appearance of the reflected images will alter. If the object viewed by reflection at the surface is fairly small, it will appear undistorted when the eye is looking along the cylinder axis meridian. As the lens is rotated, however, the image will become distorted and its size will be increased if the surface is concave and decreased if the surface is convex.

Apparatus

Box of flat astigmatic lenses; small sources of light, e.g., tungsten filament bulb (but not fluorescent strip light); crossline chart.

Procedure

(1) Position the lens so that you can see an image of a light source by reflection from the lens surface. The source should be some distance in front of you. You will, in fact, see two images of the source (one by reflection at the back of the lens). The second fainter image should be ignored.

(2) Rotate the lens, watching the image, to determine whether it changes shape. If no change can be seen the surface is spherical, and its form can be determined as explained above.

(3) If the image does alter in appearance, the surface is cylindrical. Rotate the lens until the image appears undistorted. You are now looking along the cylinder axis.

(4) With this meridian held between finger and thumb, the lens may now be held up before the crossline chart and the axis direction marked exactly by the more sensitive appearance of continuous crosslines.

If the axis marking is performed on the cylindrical surface, it will enable you to identify this surface.

(5) This is also a sensitive method of examining the quality and surface finish of a lens.

Experiment 11
TO DETERMINE THE REFRACTIVE INDEX OF A PARALLEL PLATE OF GLASS: MICROSCOPE METHOD

Theory

When an object is viewed through a plate of glass or plastics material, the image appears nearer to the object to an extent depending on the refractive index of the material. By means of a microscope the real and apparent thickness can be measured and the refractive index determined.

Apparatus

Microscope with vernier scale; thin plate of glass for the stage; parallel plate to be tested.

Procedure

A small cross is marked on the thin plate, which is fixed on the stage and carefully focused. Its position is recorded as Reading 1. The microscope is racked up sufficiently to place the parallel plate over the cross on the thin plate and again focused. The position is recorded as Reading 2. Finally the microscope is racked up to focus the top of the parallel plate and the position is recorded as Reading 3 *(Figure 11.1)*.

The experiment should be repeated at least six times, altering the position of the microscope in its housing so that different readings are obtained, and the results tabulated as follows.

Readings			*Thickness*		*n*
1	*2*	*3*	*(3) − (1) = t*	*(3) − (2) = t'*	$\dfrac{t}{t'} = n$

Conclusions

Is the method reliable? How would you apply it to a liquid?

Reading 3 →

Reading 2 →

Reading 1 →

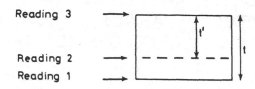

Figure 11.1. t is the real thickness of the glass block and is given by the difference between Readings 1 and 3 on the microscope vernier. t' is the apparent thickness of the glass block and is given by the difference between Readings 2 and 3 on the microscope vernier. The refractive index of the glass block
$$n = t/t'$$

Exercises

(1) Near the edge of a pond the water appears to be one metre deep. Calculate its real depth assuming the refractive index of water to be 4/3. (*Answer:* 4/3 metres.)

(2) Show that the relation $n = t/t'$ is only approximately true. Refer to *Figure 11.2.*

Proof: $n = \dfrac{\sin i}{\sin i'} = \dfrac{EB/DB}{EB/AB} = \dfrac{AB}{DB} = \dfrac{AE}{DE} = \dfrac{t}{t'}$

if the block is viewed from above so that B coincides with E.

Hence $\dfrac{\text{Real depth}}{\text{Apparent depth}} = n.$

(3) A microscope is focused upon a small object, and when the object is covered with a sheet of transparent material the microscope must be raised a distance of 2.1 mm to refocus the small object and a further distance of 4.5 mm to focus upon a mark on the upper surface of the sheet. What is the refractive index of the material of the sheet? (*Answer:* 1.467.)

(4) A block of glass rests on a sheet of paper. If the thickness of the block is 2.5 cm and its refractive index is 1.5, find the apparent displacement of the paper. (*Answer:* 0.883 cm.)

Figure 11.2. A ray AB from the object point A is refracted at the point B on the upper surface of the block and emerges in the direction BC. CB produced intersects EA at the point D. An eye viewing point A along EA sees A imaged at the point D. The refractive index n of the block is the ratio AB/DB. If the angles i and i' are small, AB and DB will be of almost the same magnitude as AE and DE respectively. Hence approximately n = AE/DE = t/t'

(5)   Why does a pond of clear water appear less deep than it really is? Find an expression for the apparent depth of a pond for perpendicular incidence and use it to find the apparent depth of a pond whose real depth is 6 m. (*Answer:* 4.5 m.)

Experiment 12
TOTAL INTERNAL REFLECTION

Theory

When a ray of light passes from glass to air it is refracted away from the normal *(Figure 12.1)*. The refractive index of glass is greater than that of air and the incident ray AC is passing from a more dense to a less dense medium. There will be an angle i such that the refracted ray CB lies along the surface of the glass so that i' is 90° *(Figure 12.2)*; the angle of incidence i is then said to be the critical angle i_c. If ray AC makes an angle of incidence with the normal greater than the critical angle, the ray AC will be totally internally reflected.

Applying the law of refraction,

$$\frac{\sin i'}{\sin i_c} = n$$

where n is the refractive index of the glass.

$$\text{But } i' = 90°$$
$$\text{and } \sin 90° = 1,$$

$$\therefore \frac{1}{\sin i_c} = n.$$

This experiment is to determine the critical angle from glass to air and hence the refractive index of the glass. The method can also be used to determine the refractive indices of liquids.

Apparatus

Drawing board, pins, semi-circular Perspex or glass block, protractor, paraffin.

Figure 12.1. Ray AC is refracted away from the normal when passing from glass into air. AC makes angle i with the normal and the refracted ray CB makes angle i' with the normal. As angle i increases, angle i' will also increase, but at a faster rate. When ray CB just lies along the surface of the glass, i.e., i' is 90°, ray AC will make an angle i_c, the critical angle, with the normal

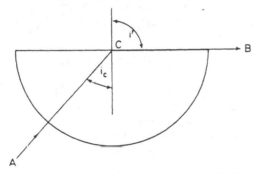

Figure 12.2. C is the centre of the semi-circular block. Hence any ray directed towards C will be normal to the curved surface. Angle i_c is the critical angle if incident ray AC is refracted so that it is coincident with the plane surface of the semi-circular block. This will occur when i' is 90° and ray CB will coincide with the plane surface

Procedure

(1) Place the semi-circular block on the sheet of paper and draw round it. Place a pin at the centre C. Then any ray directed towards C will be normal to the curved surface. Looking through the block at the pin, a clear view of the pin is obtained with the eye in a position between A and B *(Figure 12.3)*. When the head is moved, a shadow appears to cross the plane surface. When the shadow edge reaches the pin C, a pin is pushed into the paper at A so that it appears in line with C just as the shadow reaches C. This observation is repeated for the

other side of the block and position B is obtained. Remove the block and draw lines AC and CB; then angle ACB is twice the critical angle i_c.

$$\text{Hence } n = \frac{1}{\sin(ACB/2)} = \frac{1}{\sin i_c}.$$

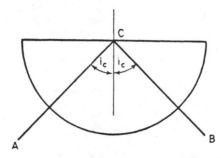

Figure 12.3

(2) Place a drop of water at C so that a water film exists between the pin and the semi-circular block. Repeat the experiment, and the critical angle i'_c for a glass/water surface can be determined. The refractive index of water n_w is given by

$$n_w = \frac{\sin i'_c}{\sin i_c}$$

(3) Repeat section (2) with paraffin and other available substances.

Exercises

(1) Prove that $n_w = \dfrac{\sin i'_c}{\sin i_c}$.

(2) The critical angle of a semi-circular glass block in air is 48° 12′. What is its refractive index? (*Answer:* 1.5.)

(3) Calculate the lowest refractive index for the glass of a right-angled prism used as a reflector to turn light through 90°.

(4) A point object is situated 6 cm below the surface of water of refractive index 4/3. What is the minimum radius of a circular card which, when floated on the surface of the water with the centre of the card directly above the point object, makes it impossible to view the point object? (*Answer:* 6.80 cm.)

Experiment 13
RULES OF TRANSPOSITION:
SPHERO-CYLINDRICAL LENSES

Theory

Two unequal cylinders A and B, placed in contact with their axes at right angles to each other, can be replaced by

(1) a sphere of power A combined with a cylinder of power $(B - A)$ with its axis parallel to the axis of cylinder B, or

(2) a sphere of power B combined with a cylinder of power $(A - B)$ with its axis parallel to the axis of cylinder A.

Thus we have three forms in which a sphero-cylindrical prescription may be written, and limiting ourselves to spherical and cylindrical surfaces only, there are three forms in which a given prescription incorporating a cylindrical component can be made up. These forms are known as the 'crossed cylinder' form and the two 'alternative sphero-cylinder' forms.

Consider the pair of cylinders $+ 1.00$ DC $\times$ 90 and $+ 3.00$ DC $\times$ 180 placed in contact with their axes in the given positions. We will describe such a pair of cylinders as follows:

$$+ 1.00 \text{ DC} \times 90 \ / + 3.00 \text{ DC} \times 180$$

and will call a prescription written as such the *cross-cyl.* form of the prescription. This form tells us immediately the powers required and also along which directions they are operative. These would be the powers found by neutralization or from a focimeter.

Applying the rules given above, we discover that this particular cross-cyl. is equivalent to

(1)   a sphere of power + 1.00 DS combined with a cylinder of power (3.00 − 1.00) + 2.00 DC, axis 180, or

(2)   a sphere of power + 3.00 DS combined with a cylinder of power (1.00 − 3.00) − 2.00 DC, axis 90; i.e.,

       (1)   + 1.00 DS / + 2.00 DC × 180, or
       (2)   + 3.00 DS / − 2.00 DC × 90,

which is the manner in which a *sphere-cylinder* prescription is usually written.

It is seen that these prescriptions are equivalent to each other. The focal properties of each lens, assumed thin, are the same. In one of the alternative *sph.-cyl.* forms of the prescription the cylinder is written with a plus sign, in the other form with a minus sign.

The rules for transposition from one form to another are as follows.

Cross-cyl. to sph.-cyl.

Sph.   =   Either cross-cyl. power written as a sphere.

Cyl.   =   Algebraic difference between the cross-cyls., i.e., the power which must be added to the cross-cyl. taken as the sphere to produce the second cross-cyl.

Axis   =   Same as axis of cross-cyl. *not* chosen as sphere.

Examples. − (1)   + 2.00 DC × 90 / + 4.00 DC × 180

           ≡ + 2.00 DS / + 2.00 DC × 180, or
           + 4.00 DS / − 2.00 DC × 90-

      (2)   − 1.00 DC × 180 / − 2.50 DC × 90

           ≡ − 1.00 DS / − 1.50 DC × 90, or
           − 2.50 DS / + 1.50 DC × 180.

It should be noted that the sphere powers in each of the sph.-cyl. forms are the same as the powers of the original cross-cyl.

Sph.-cyl. to cross-cyl.

1st cross-cyl. =   Sphere of sph.-cyl. prescription written as a cylinder with its axis at right angles to the axis of the cylinder in the sph-cyl. prescription.

2nd cross-cyl.   =   Algebraic sum of sphere and cylinder of sph.-cyl. prescription written as a cylinder with its axis the same as the axis of the sph.-cyl. prescription.

Examples. – (1)   + 1.50 DS / + 0.50 DC × 90

≡ + 1.50 DC × 180 / + 2.00 DC × 90

(2)   + 2.00 DS/ – 0.50 DC × 180

≡ + 2.00 DC × 90 / + 1.50 DC × 180

(3)   – 5.75 DS / + 2.25 DC × 90

≡ – 5.75 DC × 180 / – 3.50 DC × 90.

Alternative sph.-cyl. forms

New sph.   =   Algebraic sum of old sphere and cylinder.
New cyl.   =   Old cylinder but with sign changed.
New axis   =   At right angles to the old axis.

Examples. – (1)   + 3.00 DS / + 0.75 DC × 180

≡ + 3.75 DS / – 0.75 DC × 90

(2)   – 2.00 DS / + 3.00 DC × 90

≡ + 1.00 DS / – 3.00 DC × 180.

Exercise

Transpose the following prescriptions into their two alternative forms.

(1)   + 3.00 DC × 90 / + 7.00 DC × 180.
(2)   – 4.50 DC × 180 / – 2.25 DC × 90.
(3)   + 1.00 DC × 60 / – 1.00 DC × 150.
(4)   – 12.00 DC × 45 / – 15.00 DC × 135.
(5)   – 2.00 DS / + 1.75 DC × 20
(6)   + 4.75 DS / – 0.25 DC × 170.
(7)   – 6.25 DS / + 3.75 DC × 115.
(8)   + 0.50 DS / – 0.75 DC × 5.
(9)   – 0.75 DS / + 0.50 DC × 55.
(10)   + 11.75 DS / + 2.75 DC × 160.

Draw cross-sectional sketches of the transposed forms. *Figure 26.1a* shows a cross-sectional view of a plus spherical surface combined with a minus cylindrical surface.

Experiment 14
REFRACTIVE INDEX OF A LIQUID.
APPARENT DEPTH

Theory

An object seen through a liquid appears nearer to the surface than it actually is. The refractive index may be calculated from the formula

refractive index = real depth divided by apparent depth.

If values of real depth are plotted against corresponding values of apparent depth, the slope of the graph is the refractive index.

Apparatus

Microscope with vernier scale, beaker, liquid, lycopodium powder.

Procedure

Focus on a cross on the inside of the bottom of the empty beaker. Note the reading on the vernier scale. Alter the microscope so that the cross is out of focus. Repeat for at least two more observations. Record the three settings and their average as Reading 1. Place a little liquid in the beaker, refocus and record the settings and average as Reading 2. Place a speck of powder on the surface, focus on it, and record the settings as Reading 3.

Repeat at least six times with varying depths of liquid. Tabulate all readings as follows.

Readings			Depths	
1	2	3	Real = (3) — (1)	Apparent = (3) — (2)

Plot your results, making the graph as large as possible, and deduce the refractive index of the liquid.

Exercises

(1) Prove the statements made in the theory.

(2) A block of glass rests on a sheet of paper. The thickness of the block is 5 cm and its refractive index is 1.5. Show that the apparent displacement of the paper is 1.7 cm.

If a microscope is not available, refer to Experiment 34.

Experiment 15
NEUTRALIZATION OF
SPHERO-CYLINDRICAL LENSES — 1

Theory

The numerical power of an astigmatic lens varies from a minimum along its axis meridian (or base curve meridian in the case of a toric lens) to a maximum along its power meridian. When we have to determine the power of an astigmatic lens, we are interested only in the these minimum and maximum powers. In order to prevent confusion, therefore, it is always advisable first to mark these principal meridians on the lens and then to ensure in the transverse test that these meridians remain parallel to the limbs of the crossline chart which is being used. It might help the student to mark, in addition to the axis meridian of the lens, two short lines at the extremities of the power meridian so that he is quite sure that the transverse test is being applied along the correct meridians. With some practice he should eventually be able to dispense with these secondary markings.

Just as with spherical lenses, the crossline chart used for neutralization should be as far from the observer as possible and the lens combination should be held at full arm's length as neutralization is approached.

In this experiment we will consider how a sph.-cyl. lens may be neutralized by the use of spherical test lenses.

In order that we may completely identify a sph.-cyl. lens, it is necessary

(1) to determine which is the cylindrical surface;
(2) to determine whether this surface is convex or concave; and
(3) to locate and mark the cylinder axis.

40

Since a cylindrical surface is plane along its axis meridian, it will be realized that any power which is found along the axis meridian of the lens is due to the spherical component alone. Thus neutralization along the axis meridian produces the sphere.

Neutralization along the meridian at right angles to the cylinder axis (the power meridian of the lens) produces the sphere plus the cylinder, and by subtracting the spherical component from this second power we may determine the cylinder.

Finally, the axis direction of the cylinder may be recorded.

Examples

Powers found by neutralization		Prescription and form of lens
Along cyl. axis	Along power meridian	
+ 1.00	+ 3.00	+ 1.00 / + 2.00
− 2.50	− 1.50	− 2.50 / + 1.00
− 0.25	− 0.75	− 0.25 / − 0.50
+ 1.25	+ 0.50	+ 1.25 / − 0.75
+ 1.50	− 1.00	+ 1.50 / − 2.50

Apparatus

Flat astigmatic lenses with horizontal meridian and front surface marked; neutralizing set; crossline chart; protractor.

Procedure

(1)   By means of the straight-edge or reflection test, determine the form of the cylindrical surface and the axis direction.

(2)   Using the rotation test, accurately mark the cylinder axis as described in Experiment 7.

(3)   Neutralize the lens along the axis meridian. Record the power found by neutralization as the sphere. Before replacing the neutralizing lens, note whether the movement along the power meridian is 'with' or 'against'.

In order to prevent the combination of a series of test lenses in contact with the unknown lens, replace the lens used to neutralize the axis meridian and choose a new test lens to neutralize the power meridian.

(4) Neutralize the lens along its power meridian. This power is the sum of the sphere and the cylinder. Subtract the power of the sphere from this second power and record the result as the cylinder.

(5) With front surface uppermost, place the lens on the protractor with the marked horizontal meridian along the 180 meridian of the protractor. Record the cylinder axis direction in standard notation.

Experiment 16
NEUTRALIZATION OF
SPHERO-CYLINDRICAL LENSES – 2

Theory

In Experiment 15 we found the powers of sph.-cyl. lenses by the use of spherical trial lenses only. In this experiment we will consider how a sph.-cyl. lens may be neutralized using both spherical and cylindrical trial lenses. The advantage of using a cylindrical trial lens is that an unknown lens may be neutralized completely in the sense that when the trial lenses are in position, no apparent movement should be detected in any meridian of the combination.

It will be realised that when neutralization has been achieved, the trial sphere is neutralizing the spherical component of the unknown lens and the trial cylinder is neutralizing the cylindrical component.

We must begin as in Experiment 15 by locating and marking the cylinder axis.

Apparatus

Flat astigmatic lenses with horizontal meridian and front surface marked; neutralizing set; crossline chart; protractor.

Procedure

(1) By means of the straight-edge or reflection test, determine the cylindrical surface and the axis direction.

(2) Using the rotation test, accurately mark the cylinder axis as described in Experiment 7.

(3) Using spherical trial lenses, neutralize the lens along the axis meridian. Record the power found by neutralization as the sphere.

When the spherical component of the lens has been neutralized, note whether the movement along the power meridian is with or against.

(4) With the spherical trial lens still in position, neutralize the power meridian of the lens using appropriate plano-cylinders from the trial case—positive cyls. if the residual movement along the power meridian was found to be 'with' in step (3), held with their axes exactly parallel to the axis of the unknown lens.

(5) When the power meridian has been neutralized, apply the transverse test to other meridians of the combination to ensure that it is completely neutralized. Also apply the rotation test to verify that there is no scissors movement.

Record the power of the cylindrical trial lens — with sign changed — as the cylindrical component of the prescription.

(6) With front surface uppermost, place the lens on the protractor with the marked horizontal meridian along the 180 meridian of the protractor. Record the cylinder axis direction in standard notation.

Experiment 17
POSITIVE LENS. MEASUREMENT OF FOCAL LENGTH. CONJUGATE FOCI

Theory

The positions of an object and its image formed by a lens are connected by the following relations:

$$\frac{1}{l'} - \frac{1}{l} = \frac{1}{f'}; \quad L' - L = F; \quad F = \frac{1}{f' \text{ in metres}}$$

where l and l' are the distances in metres of object and image respectively *from* the lens. $L = \frac{1}{l}$ and $L' = \frac{1}{l'}$ are respectively the incident and emergent vergences at the lens, f' is the second focal length of the lens and F is the focal power. Vergences and powers are usually expressed in dioptres, the reciprocals of the corresponding distances in metres. Corresponding object and image positions are known as *conjugate foci (Figure 17.1)*.

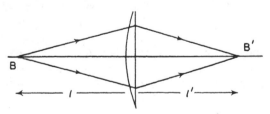

Figure 17.1. Object point B, distant l metres from the lens of surface powers F_1 and F_2, is imaged by the lens at B', distant l' metres from the lens. If the lens is thin, the total focal power $F = F_1 + F_2$ and
$$1/l' - 1/l = 1/f' = F$$

45

In substituting numerical values in the above expressions, due regard must be paid to signs. Distances measured in the direction in which the light is travelling are positive, while those against are negative. The incident light will be considered as travelling from left to right.

Apparatus

Optical bench; object; lens holder and lenses to be measured; ground glass screen.

Procedure

(1) Find the focal length roughly by using a distant lamp as an object and receiving the image on a piece of paper. The distance from the lens to the paper is roughly the focal length.

(2) Set up object, lens and screen on the bench, making the object distance appreciably more than twice the estimated focal length. Carefully focus a sharp image on the screen and note the bench reading. Repeat the setting of image screen three times and enter the mean of the three readings as the image position.

(3) Repeat the experiment at least five times with object distances both greater and less than twice the estimated focal length.

Tabulate your results as follows.

1	2	3	4	5	6	7	8
Lens No.	Positions on bench			l	l'	L	L'
	Object	Lens	Image				
38	0	60	100	-60	40	-1.67	2.5

Draw a graph, plotting L horizontally and L' vertically. Deduce the value of F from the graph.

Draw a graph, plotting l horizontally and l' vertically, and deduce the values of f and f'.

Exercises

(1) A positive lens has a focal length of 30 cm. Find the position of the image when an object is situated (a) 80 cm and (b) 10 cm from the lens. (*Answer:* (a) $+48$ cm real image; (b) -15 cm virtual image.)

(2)   When an object was placed 40 cm in front of a lens, a virtual image was formed 50 cm in front of the lens. What was the focal power of the lens? (*Answer:* + 0.50 D.)

Use of conjugate foci relationships

A few examples are given below to illustrate the use of the conjugate foci relationships.

(1)   A real object is placed 25 cm from a thin lens whose surface powers are respectively + 3 D and + 5 D. Find the position of the image.

> *Answer:* Light is travelling from left to right. The object is 25 cm from the thin lens, which has surface powers $F_1 = + 3$ D, $F_2 = + 5$ D. We are required to find the position of the image.
>
> $l = -25$ cm (since all distances are measured *from* the lens and distances measured in an opposite direction to that of the direction of the light are negative) or -0.25 metre.
> Hence the object vergence L is

$$\frac{1}{-0.25} = -4 \text{ D.}$$

The total focal power F of a thin lens with surface powers F_1 and F_2 is given by $F = F_1 + F_2$.

Hence $F = + 3$ D $+ 5$ D $= + 8$ D
$L' - L = F.$

Hence $L' - (-4 \text{ D}) = + 8$ D
$L' + 4$ D $= + 8$ D
$L' = + 8$ D $- 4$ D $= + 4$ D.

Hence $l' = + 0.25$ metre or $+ 25$ cm. Since l' is positive, a real image is formed 25 cm beyond the lens.

Figure 17.2

(2) A plano-convex lens has a radius of curvature of + 5 cm and refractive index 1.5. Find the focal power of the lens.

An object is placed 12.5 cm from the lens. Find the position of the image *(Figure 17.2)*.

Answer: The focal power of the lens surface in the diagram is given by $F = \dfrac{n-1}{r}$ where r is in metres and F is in dioptres of focal power.

Hence r = + 0.5 metre, since r is measured from the lens surface to the centre of curvature and is positive in the example.

Then $F = \dfrac{n-1}{r}$

$\quad = \dfrac{1.5-1}{0.5}$

$\quad = + 10 \text{ D.}$

$l = -12.5 \text{ cm.}$

hence $L = -8 \text{ D}$
$$L' - L = F$$
$$L' - (-8) = + 10$$
$$L' + 8 = + 10$$
$$L' = + 2 \text{ D}$$
$$l' = + 0.5 \text{ metre or 50 cm.}$$

Hence a real image is formed 50 cm beyond the lens.

Figure 17.3

(3) A biconvex lens has radii of curvature of magnitude 10 cm and 12.5 cm and refractive index 1.5. An object is placed 20 cm from the lens. Find the position of the image.

Answer: Referring to *Figure 17.3,*

$$r_1 = +10 \text{ cm, and}$$
$$r_2 = -12.5 \text{ cm.}$$

r_2 is negative since it is measured from the second surface to the centre of curvature, which is opposite to the direction of the light.

If we consider that light always travels from left to right, then distances measured from the lens surface to the left are negative and distances measured from the lens surface to the right are positive.

The biconvex lens has surface powers F_1 and F_2, and

$$F_1 = \frac{n-1}{r}, \quad F_2 = \frac{1-n}{r_2}$$

$$F_1 = \frac{1.5 - 1}{0.1} = +5 \text{ D}$$

$$F_2 = \frac{1 - 1.5}{-0.125} = \frac{0.5}{0.125} = +4 \text{ D.}$$

If the lens is assumed thin, $F = F_1 + F_2$.

Hence $F = +5 \text{ D} + 4 \text{ D} = +9 \text{ D}$

$l = -20$ cm, hence $L = -5 \text{ D}$

$$L' - L = F$$
$$L' - (-5 \text{ D}) = +9 \text{ D}$$
$$L' + 5 \text{ D} = +9 \text{ D}$$
$$L' = +4 \text{ D.}$$

Hence $l' = +25$ cm, therefore a real image is formed 25 cm beyond the lens.

Experiment 18
NEGATIVE LENS. MEASUREMENT OF
FOCAL LENGTH. CONJUGATE FOCI

Theory

In Experiment 17 it was established that for a positive lens,

$$\frac{1}{f'} = \frac{1}{l'} - \frac{1}{l} \text{ or } F = L' - L.$$

The object of this experiment is to show that these formulae hold for negative lenses and to determine the focal power of a negative lens.

Since such a lens will not form a real image of a real object, it is necessary to use an auxiliary positive lens A_1 which forms a real image B_1 of the object O. This image B_1 acts as a *virtual object* for the negative lens A_2. The light converging towards B_1 is rendered less convergent by the lens A_2 and converges to a more distant image B'_1. Then for the negative lens A_2, the object distance is $A_2 B_1$ and the image distance is $A_2 B'_1$ *(Figure 18.1)*.

The same method may be used also in measuring the power of a weak positive lens which would not give a real image of a real object within the range of the optical bench.

Apparatus

Optical bench, positive lens, negative and weak positive lens to be measured, object, screen.

Procedure

Set up object O, positive lens A_1 and screen and obtain a sharp image of the object on the screen; note this position B_1. Place the negative lens A_2 between the positive lens and screen and move the screen back until a sharp image is again obtained, at position B'_1. Position the screen three times and note the mean position B'_1. Tabulate the results.

Repeat the experiment with the negative lens in various positions. Move the positive lens to a new position and repeat the experiment. Use the same method to measure the weak positive lens.

Record your results as follows.

O	A_1	A_2	B_1	B'_1	l	l'	L	L'	F_2	f'_2

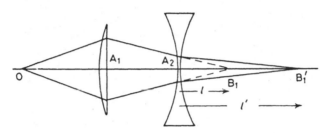

Figure 18.1. The auxiliary positive lens, focal power F_1, forms an image at B_1 of the object at O. The negative lens, focal power F_2, is placed as shown and image B_1 is now a virtual object for the negative lens. The convergent light incident on the negative lens is rendered less convergent by the negative lens and a real image is formed at B'_1. Let A_1 and A_2 be the positions on the optical bench of the positive and negative lenses respectively. Then the object distance for the negative lens is given by distance A_2B_1 and the image distance by $A_2B'_1$. Let $A_2B'_1 = l'$ and $A_2B_1 = l$. Then $1/l' - 1/l = F_2$ where l' and l are expressed in metres and F_2 is the focal power in dioptres of the negative lens

Exercises

(1) In certain positions of the negative lens no real image can be obtained. Why is this?

(2) An object is placed 1 metre in front of a positive lens of 50 cm focal length, and a negative lens of 25 cm focal length is placed 75 cm behind the positive lens. Find the position of the final image. (*Answer:* infinity.)

(3) If the object in exercise (2) were moved to infinity, where would the negative lens have to be placed so that the final image was

still at infinity? What kind of optical system would the lenses then form?

(4)   Draw a graph, plotting L horizontally and L' vertically. Deduce the value of F.

(5)   Draw a graph, plotting l horizontally and l' vertically. Deduce the values of f and f'.

Experiment 19
THE PRINCIPLE OF THE LENS
MEASURE – 1

Theory

The lens measure is a form of spherometer. The spherometer is an instrument used to measure the radius of curvature of a curved surface.

In *Figure 19.1*, BAD is a trace of a spherical surface of radius OD. AC is termed the sagitta or sag of the curve for a given length of chord BD.

Let BD = 2y
   AC = s
   OD = r.

Then in the right-angled triangle OCD,

$$OD^2 = CD^2 + OC^2$$
$$r^2 = y^2 + (r - s)^2,$$
$$\text{which reduces to } 2rs = y^2 + s^2$$
$$\text{or } r = \frac{y^2}{2s} + \frac{s}{2} \qquad \dots (1)$$

The spherometer measures the sag s for a given chord 2y and hence r can be calculated from equation 1. When the distance s is small compared with y then the term $\frac{s}{2}$ is very small compared with $\frac{y^2}{2s}$.

Then $r = \frac{y^2}{2s}$

which is an approximation.

In ophthalmic lens work, s is usually small compared with y and hence the approximate relationship is used. This experiment is to

53

compare equations (1) and (2) and to find the error introduced by using the approximation.

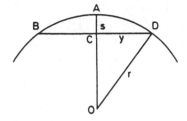

Figure 19.1. The sag formula. BAD is the trace of a spherical surface of centre O and radius OD = r. BD is a chord of length 2y (CD = y). AC is the sagitta or sag of the surface s for the chord 2y. In the right-angled triangle OCD, $OD^2 = CD^2 + OC^2$, or $r^2 = y^2 + (r-s)^2$, or $r^2 - 2rs + y^2 = 0$

Apparatus

Drawing board, paper, compasses, ruler.

Procedure

Draw the largest possible semi-circle, centre O *(Figure 19.1)*. Draw various chords of diameter 2y corresponding to sags AC having values of 5 mm, 10 mm, 20 mm, 40 mm and 80 mm. In each case measure the length 2y. Measure on the paper the radius OD. Calculate the radius using equations (1) and (2).

Calculate the percentage error introduced by using the relationship $r = \dfrac{y^2}{2s}$. This can be done in the following manner:

Let r be the radius obtained using equation (1).
Let r_a be the radius (approximate) obtained using equation (2).
The percentage error is given by $\dfrac{(r - r_a)}{r} \times 100$.

Record your results as follows.

s	y	$\dfrac{y^2}{2s}$	$\dfrac{s}{2}$	Radius by calculation		Error (per cent)	Radius measured directly
				Exact	Approx.		

Exercises

Draw a graph plotting the sag s horizontally and the corresponding percentage error vertically. From the graph read off the percentage errors corresponding to sags of 30 mm and 60 mm. Verify these values by calculation using equations (1) and (2).

Example. – If a lens measure is calibrated using the relationship $r = \dfrac{y^2}{2s}$, will it be more accurate for steep surfaces or shallow surfaces? Give reasons for your answer.

Notes on the graph

The true value of r is given by

$$r = \frac{BC^2}{2AC} + \frac{AC}{2}$$

The approximate value of r_a is given by

$$r_a = \frac{BC^2}{2AC}$$

The difference between these two values is $\dfrac{AC}{2}$

The percentage error is then given by

$$\frac{\dfrac{AC}{2}}{\dfrac{BC^2}{2AC} + \dfrac{AC}{2}} \times 100$$

$$= \frac{\dfrac{s}{2}}{r\ (exact)} \times 100$$

$$= \frac{50s}{r}$$

Hence a graph of percentage error plotted vertically and sag horizontally will give a straight line whose slope has a value of $\dfrac{50}{r}$ and which goes through the origin.

Experiment 20
THE PRINCIPLE OF THE LENS
MEASURE — 2

Theory

Figure 20.1 illustrates the principle of the optician's lens measure. A and C are fixed points midway between which is the moving point B. A plane surface placed against the points A, B, C of the lens measure will depress the point B so that A, B and C are level. The movement of the arm BD will cause the pointer centred at O to rotate and come to rest at the zero position of the scale if the instrument is accurate. If the instrument is now placed on a curved surface, the central point B will move a distance s. The distance between the fixed points A and C is 2y. In an actual instrument the lever mechanism is more complicated than illustrated. The focal power of an optical surface in air F is given by

$$F = \frac{(n-1)}{r} \qquad \ldots (1)$$

F is in dioptres, r is in metres, and n is the refractive index.
In the previous experiment it was shown that

$$r = \frac{y^2}{2s} \text{ approximately} \qquad \ldots (2)$$

From equations (1) and (2),

$$F = \frac{(n-1)\,2s}{y^2}.$$

y is a constant of the instrument.

n is the refractive index of spectacle glass, hence F is proportional to the sag s. The scale of the lens measure is calibrated to read focal power and is approximately uniform.

Since the three points of the lens measure lie in a straight line, it can be used to measure the curvature of the principal meridians of a toroidal or cylindrical surface.

Care must be taken in any measurement that the instrument is perpendicular to the surface.

Figure 20.1. A and C are the two fixed legs of the instrument. B is the movable leg which actuates the mechanism causing the pointer to rotate. (The lever mechanism is more complicated in practice than that shown.) The distance AC is 2y. The height of point B above or below the straight line joining points A and C represents the sag s measured by the instrument

Apparatus

Neutralizing set and crossline chart; lens measure; plane surface; toric lenses; protractor.

Procedure

(1) Check the zero reading of the lens measure on the plane surface. Reset if necessary so that the point indicates zero. If this is not possible, record the zero error, e.g., if the instrument reads − 0.75 DS on the plane surface record the zero error as − 0.75 sph.

(2) Using the crossline chart, mark on the lens the principal meridians.

(3) Place the points of the lens measure carefully along one of the principal meridians and obtain a reading.

(4) Withdraw the points of the lens measure from the surface, rotate the lens measure through 90 degrees and obtain a reading for the other meridian. Do not rotate the lens measure while it is in contact with the surface of the lens.

(5) Estimate the positive cylinder axis direction if the lens is edged or has a horizontal datum line.

(6) Record your results for all the lenses as indicated, then verify by neutralization and the lens setting protractor.

(7) Compare the results of the lens measure and neutralization.
Tabulate your results as follows.

Lens No.	Lens measure readings		Corrected lens measure readings zero error			Neutralization		
	1st meridian	2nd meridian	1st meridian	2nd meridian	Estimated axis	Sph.	Cyl.	Axis

Experiment 21
TO DETERMINE THE REFRACTIVE
INDEX OF A LENS

Theory

It is sometimes necessary to determine the refractive index of a lens without destroying the form of the lens.

Since the power (F) of a lens is equal to $(n - 1)(R_1 - R_2)$, if the values of F, R_1, R_2 are known, the value of the refractive index (n) can be calculated.

Apparatus

Optical bench, spherometer, lenses.

Procedure

By means of the spherometer, determine the curvature of the lens surfaces R_1 and R_2. Determine the focal power of the lens on the optical bench. From this calculate the refractive index of the lens.

Record your results as follows.

R_1	R_2	F	n

Conclusions

State the practical uses of this experiment.

Exercises

(1) The radius of curvature of a plano convex lens is 6.25 cm and its focal length is 12.5 cm. Calculate its refractive index. (*Answer:* 1.5.)

(2) A positive lens of focal length 25 cm has a refractive index of 1.5. The radius of curvature of the front surface is + 5 cm. What will be the radius of the second surface? What is the form of the lens? (*Answer:* + 8.33 cm).

Experiment 22
THE AXIS DIRECTION OF ASTIGMATIC LENSES: STANDARD NOTATION

Theory

The axis direction of an astigmatic lens is always specified in standard notation, and this notation should be thoroughly mastered by the student.

Imagine that you are looking at somebody's face. His right eye lies on your left hand side and his left eye lies on your right-hand side. The eyes are invariably shown in this position in diagrams *(Figure 22.1)*. A horizontal line drawn through the eye represents the zero meridian for standard notation.

The axis direction is specified in degrees commencing with 0 on the right side of each eye and numbering anti-clockwise round to 180 on the left.

The notation then renumbers below the horizontal meridian, again beginning with 0, and passes back to its origin where it becomes 180. The origin lies at the nasal side (marked N in *Figure 22.1*) of the right eye but at the temporal side (marked T in *Figure 22.1*) of the left eye.

The horizontal meridian is never referred to as the 0 meridian but always as the 180 meridian. The vertical meridian is referred to as the 90 meridian. The notation is usually expressed in 5 degree stages, but occasionally 2½ or even 1 degree stages are prescribed.

The degrees sign itself is always omitted. This is a safeguard against such errors as a carelessly written 5° being mistaken for 50, etc. Most optical protractors — those used for marking and setting spectacle lenses — are numbered in standard notation. Occasionally, however, the student might come across a protractor which bears reversed standard notation. These are often called 'reversed protractors' and are used in surfacing instruction. The utmost care must be exercised if the protractor is reversed, for it only reads in standard notation if the lens is laid with its front surface downwards upon the protractor.

Figure 22.1. Standard axis notation. The notation commences on the right-hand side of each lens and numbers anti-clockwise to 180. It then renumbers below the 180 meridian, 180 becoming zero. The notation is the same for each eye

Figure 22.2. Examples of standard axis notation

When the axis direction of an astigmatic lens is to be recorded, the student should make sure that he is looking at the front surface of the lens and then estimate the position of the axis in relation to the horizontal or 180 meridian of the lens before checking the result on the protractor. If he adopts this safeguard he is far less likely to misread standard notation.

Figure 22.2 shows some lenses with their axes marked. The axis directions accompanying each lens should be verified.

Experiment 23
AXIS MARKING AND SETTING

Theory

The process of marking and setting a spectacle lens before it enters the glazing department for cutting and edging is called *laying off.* The purpose of laying off is to inform the glazing department of the correct orientation of the lens so that they can concentrate on the necessary edging and fitting of the lens into its mount. The glazing department require just four details:

(1) Which eye the lens is intended for.
(2) Which is the front surface of the lens.
(3) The orientation of the cylinder axis.
(4) The position of the optical centre.

All this information is provided by the laying-off section of the prescription house, who convey each detail to the glazing department by suitably marking the lens. In this experiment we will assume that the optical centre of the lens is to be located at the standard optical centre position. This position is the point at which the prescription house places the optical centres of its lenses when no decentration or prismatic effect has been called for. The position always lies on the vertical line which passes through the datum centre, but its actual height depends upon the particular prescription house.

The first step of the laying-off process is to ensure that the lens has the prescribed power and form. This is performed by neutralization and by the lens measure. The axis of the lens is then marked, together with the optical centre. After this the lens is laid upon the protractor with its front surface uppermost and the cylinder axis placed along the correct meridian. The lens is now shifted until its optical centre lies at the intersection of the 90 and 180 meridians at the centre of the protractor. Finally the lens is marked with waterproof paint as shown in *Figure 23.1a* if it is for the right eye or *Figure 23.1b* if for the left

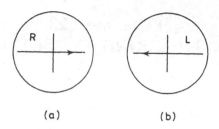

(a)   (b)

Figure 23.1. Laying off lenses for glazing

eye. The R and L indicate for which eye the lens is to be used, the small arrowhead indicating the nasal side of the lens. The marking is always performed on the front surface of the lens. The glazing department will arrange that the horizontal cutting line lies parallel to the datum line of the frame (if the standard optical centre position lies at the datum centre, the horizontal line will coincide with the datum line) and that the vertical cutting line coincides with the vertical line which bisects the datum line.

Apparatus

Box of uncut lenses together with a written prescription for each lens; centring machine, protractor, neutralizing set; waterproof ink and brush or pen, or grease pencil (for practice use).

Procedure

(1)   Sort out the lenses by neutralization to match the individual prescription forms. If necessary, check the form of each lens by lens measure.

(2)   Locate and mark the cylinder axis, which corresponds with the axis on the order form and the optical centre. (With bent lenses it is easier to view and mark the axis and centre through the concave surface of the lens.)

(3)   Lay the uncut lens on the protractor with its front surface uppermost, and rotate it until the axis on the lens lies along the prescribed meridian. Adjust the lens at the same time until its optical

centre coincides with the intersection of the 90 and 180 meridians at the centre of the protractor.

(4)   Using waterproof ink, draw a thin straight cutting line along the horizontal meridian of the lens following the 180 meridian of the protractor. This line should pass through the optical centre *(Figure 23.2a)*.

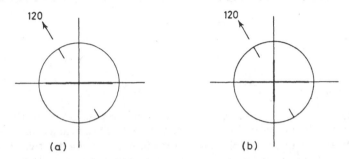

Figure 23.2.(a) Place lens on protractor with front surface upper-most and optical centre over intersection of crossline. Rotate the lens until the cylinder axis corresponds with the required meridian (120). Draw the horizontal cutting line. (b) Draw a shorter vertical line

(5)   Draw a shorter vertical line along the vertical meridian of the lens through the optical centre following the 90 meridian of the protractor *(Figure 23.2b)*.

(6)   Indicate which eye the lens is intended for by marking R or L in the upper temporal quadrant of the lens and by drawing an arrow-head near the nasal end of the horizontal cutting line as shown in *Figure 23.1*.

Experiment 24
POSITIVE LENS. MEASUREMENT OF
FOCAL LENGTH. AUTO-COLLIMATION

Theory

When a small source of light is placed at the principal focus of a convex lens, the light emerges from the lens as a parallel beam, and if the beam is reflected normally at a plane mirror it will return along its original path. This provides a simple method of determining the principal focus of a lens. This experiment illustrates the principle of auto-collimation.

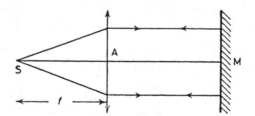

Figure 24.1. Principle of auto-collimation. Light from the source S is refracted by the lens and then reflected by the mirror to undergo another refraction at the lens. If the source is at the focal point of the lens, the light is parallel after refraction by the lens. The reflected light is parallel and will be focused at S. Hence an image arises in the plane of the source S. The distance of the source from the lens will be the focal length of the lens

Apparatus

Optical bench, small source, lens to be tested, plane mirror, half screen, three lens holders.

Procedure

(1)   Set up source, lens and mirror as in *Figure 24.1* and move lens until an image of the source is formed in the plane of the source.

Record positions S, A and M and determine focal length. Verify the results by the conjugate foci method, tabulating all readings obtained.

(2)   If an optical bench is not available, the lens can be placed in contact with the plane mirror, which is placed on a flat surface. A pin is held vertically above the combination by a clamp. With the eye above the pin, an image of the pin formed by the lens/plane mirror combination and the actual pin will be seen. The height of the pin is varied until, by parallax, the object and the image are the same distance from the lens. This distance is then the focal length of the lens.

Experiment 25
NEGATIVE LENS. MEASUREMENT OF
FOCAL LENGTH. AUTO-COLLIMATION

Theory

The principle of this experiment is the same as that of Experiment 24. Divergent light from the negative lens is rendered parallel by a positive lens placed so that its first principal focus is in the position of the virtual image formed by the negative lens. This parallel light falls normally on a plane mirror and is reflected back along its original path, a real image being formed in the plane of the object.

For the negative lens we have

$$A_1 B = l, \quad A_1 B' = l'$$

$$\text{and } \frac{1}{l'} - \frac{1}{l} = \frac{1}{f'}, \text{ or } L' - L = F.$$

Apparatus

Optical bench, object, positive and negative lenses, plane mirror.

Procedure

Set up object, positive lens and mirror as in *Figure 25.1* and find the principal focus of the positive lens by the method of Experiment 24. Place the negative lens between the positive lens and the object and move the object back until a sharp image is formed in the plane of the object.

Note. – Care must be taken that the image found is not due to reflection from the concave surface of the negative lens. Repeat the experiment in a number of different positions on the bench.

				Positions on bench						
B	B'	A_1	A_2	M	l	l'	L	L'	F	f'

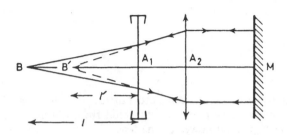

Figure 25.1. Object point B is imaged by the negative lens A_1 as a virtual image B'. If B' coincides with the focal point of positive lens A_2, the emergent light from A_2 will be parallel. This will be reflected at mirror M and an image of the point B will be imaged in the plane of B

Exercises

(1) A − 5 D lens is placed 3.33 cm in front of a + 10 D lens. How far from the negative lens must an object be placed in order that light may emerge parallel from the positive lens? (*Answer:* 10 cm.)

(2) Parallel light falls on a +2 D lens. Where must a − 8 D lens be placed in order that the light leaving the system shall be still parallel? Of what instrument is this the principle? (*Answer:* 37.5 cm from positive lens.)

Experiment 26
TORIC LENSES. TORIC TRANSPOSITION

Theory

When a thin spherical lens is bent into a different form, whatever power is added to one surface must be subtracted from the other in order to retain the correct total power of the lens. Thus a + 5.00 DS in plano-convex form has surface powers + 5.00 D and 0.00 D. If the same power is to be obtained in a curved form with a + 10.00 D surface, the other surface of the lens must be made − 5.00 D, i.e., + 5.00 has been added to the front surface and − 5.00 to the back.

Consider the sphero-cylinder + 5.00 DS/ − 2.00 DC × 90. The form of the lens is shown in *Figure 26.1a*. The surface powers are + 5.00 DS and 0.00 DC × 180/ − 2.00 DC × 90. If we were to add + 5.00 D to the spherical surface and − 5.00 D to the cylindrical surface, we would obtain surface powers + 10.00 DS and − 5.00 DC × 180/ − 7.00 DC × 90 *(Figure 26.1b)*. The curved cylindrical surface is called a *toroidal surface* and the lens has become a *toric lens*.

The toroidal surface has two principal curves. The lower numerical curve on the surface is called the *base curve* and the higher numerical curve is called the *cross curve*. A toric lens is defined as a lens which incorporates a toroidal surface and at the same time is curved in form (i.e., one surface is convex and the other concave). The toroidal surface may be convex or concave. Occasionally a 'capstan' or 'mixed' toroidal surface will be met *(Figure 26.2)*. With such a surface the base curve is taken to be the convex curve whether this is numerically higher or lower than the concave curve.

The surface powers of the toric lens shown in *Figure 26.1b* may be written as follows:

$$\frac{+\ 10.00\ \text{DS}}{-\ 5.00\ \text{DC} \ \times\ 180/\ -7.00\ \text{DC}\ \times 90}$$

and it will be appreciated that the algebraic sum of the base curve and the spherical curve (sph. curve) is the spherical component of the lens, whereas the difference between the base curve and the cross curve is the cylindrical component of the lens.

(a)   (b)

Figure 26.1.(a) Cross-sectional view of principal meridians of sphero-cylindrical lens + 5.00 DS/ − 2.00 DC x 90. The front surface power is + 5.00 DS and the back surface power is − 2.00 DC x 90. (b) Cross-sectional view of principal meridians of − 5.00 D base toric lens + 5.00 DS/ − 2.00 DC x 90. The front surface power or sphere curve is + 10.00 DS; the back surface power is − 5.00 DC x 180/ − 7.00 DC x 90; − 5.00 DC x 180 is the base curve; and − 7.00 DC x 90 is the cross curve

Figure 26.2. Capstan formation toroidal surface. The convex curve is taken to be the base curve

We could alter any one of these three surface powers provided that an equivalent alteration were made to the other two curves. Thus we could add + 11.00 D to each power of the toroidal surface, in which case we would have to add − 11.00 D to the spherical surface. The resulting surface powers would be

$$\frac{- 1.00 \text{ DS}}{+ 6.00 \text{ DS} \times 180/ + 4.00 \text{ DC} \times 90}$$

or, by a more conventional method in which the front surface power is written above the line with the base curve first,

$$\frac{+4.00 \text{ DC} \times 90/ + 6.00 \text{ DC} \times 180}{-1.00 \text{ DS}}$$

This lens would be described as a + 4.00 D base toric.

Toric transposition

The rules for transposing a given prescription into toric form if the base curve is specified are as follows. The prescription is assumed to be in one of its alternative sph.-cyl. forms.

(1) Transpose the sph.-cyl. prescription to the form which has a cylinder sign the same as that of the given base curve.

(2) Write the base curve as a cylinder with its axis at right angles to the axis of the cylindrical component of the sph.-cyl. prescription obtained after transposition in step (1).

(3) Add the cylindrical component of the sph.-cyl. prescription to the base curve to obtain the cross curve, and write this as a cylinder with its axis the same as the axis of the sph.-cyl. prescription.

(4) Subtract the base curve from the sphere of the sph.-cyl. prescription to obtain the sphere curve.

We may summarize these rules as follows.

The toric form is: $\dfrac{\text{Base curve/Cross curve}}{\text{Sph. curve}}$

and assuming that the cylinder of the sph.-cyl. prescription has the same sign as the base curve, we can write:

Base curve is given.
Cross curve = base curve + cyl. component.
Sphere curve = sphere component − base curve.

To transpose back from the toric form to sph.-cyl. form,

Sphere = base curve + sphere curve.
Cylinder = cross curve − base curve.
Axis is same as axis of cross curve.

If we have to transpose a sph.-cyl. prescription into toric form with a specified sphere curve, the rules are as follows.

TORIC LENSES. TORIC TRANSPOSITION

(1) Transpose the sph.-cyl. prescription to the form which has its cylinder sign the same as that of the base curve. This form will usually be the one in which the cylinder sign is opposite to that of the specified sphere curve.

(2) Subtract the sphere curve from the sph. component of the prescription to obtain the base curve. This is written as a cylinder with its axis at right angles to the axis of the cylindrical component of the sph.-cyl. prescription.

(3) Add the cylinder to the base curve to obtain the cross curve, whose axis will be the same as the axis of the sph.-cyl. prescription.

In short, sphere curve given:

Base curve = Sphere component − sphere curve.
Cross curve = Base curve + cyl. component.

Examples

The following examples should be carefully worked through. In each case the two alternative sph.-cyl. forms of the prescription are given together with four toric forms on ±6.00 D base curves and ±6.00 D sphere curves.

(1) + 1.00 DS/ + 2.00 DC × 90
     + 3.00 DS/ − 2.00 DC × 180

$$\frac{+ 6.00 \text{ DC} \times 180/ + 8.00 \text{ DC} \times 90}{- 5.00 \text{ DS}}$$
$$\frac{+ 9.00 \text{ DS}}{- 6.00 \text{ DC} \times 90/ - 8.00 \text{ DC} \times 180}$$

$$\frac{+ 6.00 \text{ DS}}{- 3.00 \text{ DC} \times 90/ - 5.00 \text{ DC} \times 180}$$
$$\frac{+ 7.00 \text{ DC} \times 180/ + 9.00 \text{ DC} \times 90}{- 6.00 \text{ DS}}$$

(2) − 4.50 DS/ − 0.50 DC × 45
     − 5.00 DS/ + 0.50 DC × 135

$$\frac{+ 6.00 \text{ DC} \times 45/ + 6.50 \text{ DC} \times 135}{- 11.00 \text{ DS}}$$
$$\frac{+ 1.50 \text{ DS}}{- 6.00 \text{ DC} \times 135/ - 6.50 \text{ DC} \times 45}$$

$$\frac{+ 6.00 \text{ DS}}{- 10.50 \text{ DC} \times 135/ - 11.00 \text{ DC} \times 45}$$
$$\frac{+ 1.00 \text{ DC} \times 45/ + 1.50 \text{ DC} \times 135}{- 6.00 \text{ DS}}$$

73

(3)   − 1.75 DS/ + 2.50 DC × 30
      + 0.75 DS/ − 2.50 DC × 120

$$\frac{+ 6.00\ DC \times 120/ + 8.50\ DC \times 30}{− 7.75\ DS}$$

$$\frac{+ 6.75\ DS}{− 6.00\ DC \times 30/ − 8.50\ DC \times 120}$$

$$\frac{+ 6.00\ DS}{− 5.25\ DC \times 30/ − 7.75\ DC \times 120}$$

$$\frac{+ 4.25\ DC \times 120/ + 6.75\ DC \times 30}{− 6.00\ DS}$$

(4)   + 1.00 DS/ − 8.00 DC × 5
      − 7.00 DS/ + 8.00 DC × 95

$$\frac{+ 6.00\ DC \times 5/ + 14.00\ DC \times 95}{− 13.00\ DS}$$

$$\frac{+ 7.00\ DS}{− 6.00\ DC \times 95/ − 14.00\ DC \times 5}$$

$$\frac{+ 6.00\ DS}{− 5.00\ DC \times 95/ − 13.00\ DC \times 5}$$

$$\frac{+ 7.00\ DC \times 95/ − 1.00\ DC \times 5}{− 6.00\ DS}$$

This last example requires the use of a mixed toroidal surface. It is interesting to note that there is a second toric form with a + 6.00 D base curve which also incorporates a mixed surface. This form is

$$\frac{+ 6.00\ DC \times 95/ − 2.00\ DC \times 5}{− 5.00\ DS}$$

and it should be remembered that when a prescription is to be transposed to toric form with a positive base curve, two different forms (one incorporating a mixed surface) are possible when the base curve is of smaller power than the cylinder in the sph.-cyl. prescription.

Experiment 27
NEUTRALIZATION OF TORIC LENSES

Theory

Owing to the curved surfaces of a toric lens, the straight-edge and reflection tests cannot be applied as a means of determining the base curve meridian of a toric lens, and the determination of the lens form — i.e., whether the convex surface or the concave surface is toroidal — requires the use of a lens measure. By means of the lens measure we can immediately determine which is the toroidal surface and, at the same time, record the power and position of the base curve. When these have been found, the lens may be neutralized and its surface powers recorded as shown in Experiment 26.

Apparatus

Edged toric lenses with horizontal meridian marked; neutralizing set; crossline chart; lens measure; protractor.

Procedure

(1)   By means of the lens measure, determine which is the toroidal surface by lightly rotating the measure over each surface. Record the power of the base curve and note the position of this meridian.

(2)   Hold the lens before the crossline chart with the concave surface towards the eye and by means of the rotation test accurately mark the axis direction along the base curve meridian.

(3)   Neutralize the lens along the base curve meridian. Record the power found by neutralization as the sphere.

(4)   Neutralize the lens along the cross curve meridian (i.e., at right angles to the base meridian). Record this power as the sphere plus the

cylinder. Subtract the power of the sphere from this second power and record the result as the cylinder.

(5) With front surface uppermost, place the lens on the protractor with the marked horizontal meridian along the 180 meridian of the protractor. Record the base curve direction as the cylinder axis in standard notation.

(6) When the principal powers and axis directions are known, the prescription of the lens may be written in its toric form. Write the base curve as a cylinder with its axis at right angles to the axis direction found in step (5). Add the cylindrical component of the sph.-cyl. to the base curve to obtain the cross curve and write as a cylinder with its axis the same as given in step (5). Finally subtract the base curve from the spherical component of the sph.-cyl. prescription to obtain the sphere curve.

(7.) Check the surface powers obtained in step (6) by means of the lens measure.

Record your results as shown in the table below.

Base curve (by lens measure)	Powers by neutralization		Axis (base curve)	Sph.-cyl. prescription	Toric form of prescription
	Along base	Along cross			
+ 6.00	+ 2.00	+ 3.00	30	+ 2.00/ + 1.00 × 30	+ 6.00 DC × 120/ + 7.00 DC × 30 −4.00 DS

Experiment 28
MEASUREMENT OF THE RADIUS OF
CURVATURE OF A MIRROR

Theory

Figure 28.1 shows a source S, a convex lens, and a convex mirror whose vertex is at position A.

Light from the source S after refraction by the lens is converging to form an image of the source. If this image coincides with position A so that it is formed on the vertex of the mirror, the light will return along its original path. If the convex mirror is moved towards the lens so that the centre of curvature of the mirror coincides with position A, light will again return along its original path. The distance between these two positions of the mirror is the radius of curvature of the mirror.

Apparatus

Source, convex lens, ground glass screen, convex and concave mirrors to be measured, optical bench.

Procedure

Convex mirror

(1)   Place the source, convex lens and ground glass screen on the optical bench.

(2)   Obtain an image of the source on the ground glass screen, positioning the lens so that a large image distance is obtained.

(3)   Remove the ground glass screen and place the convex mirror in the same position. An image of the source should be formed at S in the plane of the source, but it is usually very faint. Record the position A of the mirror.

(4) The convex mirror is moved towards the lens until a sharp image is formed in the plane of the source. Let this be position B of the mirror, and record it. The previous position A is now at the centre of curvature of the mirror and the distance AB moved by the mirror is the radius of curvature.

Vary the position of A and obtain at least five readings.

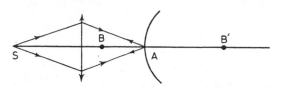

Figure 28.1. Light from source S is imaged by the lens at the intersection of the curved surface A and the optical axis. Let the curved surface represent a mirror whose radius of curvature is of magnitude BA. With the mirror at A, light will be returned along its own path. If the convex mirror is moved forward a distance equal to its radius of curvature, light will again be returned along its own path and an image of the source will be formed coincident with the source. If the mirror is concave, it is moved away from the lens to position B' where distance AB' is the radius of curvature of the concave mirror

Concave mirror

Proceed as in steps (1), (2) and (3) above.

(4) The concave mirror is moved away from the lens until a sharp image is formed in the plane of the source, position B' of the mirror, then distance AB' is the radius of curvature of the concave mirror.

Vary the position of A and obtain at least five readings.

Record your results as follows and obtain a mean reading.

Convex			Concave		
Position A	Position B	AB = r	Position A	Position B'	AB' = r

This method of determining the radius of curvature is known as Drysdale's method. It also illustrates the principle of the radiuscope, an instrument for measuring the radius of curvature of a contact lens. In this instrument the convex lens is replaced by a microscope objective and the objective is moved while the contact lens remains stationary. The movement of the microscope objective is measured by an accurate vernier scale.

Experiment 29
NEUTRALIZATION OF GLAZED LENSES

Theory

The neutralization of lenses which are glazed to spectacle frames is exactly the same as the neutralization of single lenses except that owing to the presence, of the sides of the spectacle frame, the axis direction cannot be read from a protractor in the normal fashion. Here the frame must be placed over the protractor with its front surface facing downwards so that the axis direction, which is read from a protractor calibrated in standard notation, is in fact the supplement of the true axis direction. In order to record the axis direction in standard notation, the axis indicated by the protractor must be subtracted from 180.

Apparatus

Set of glazed frames; neutralizing set; centring machine or crossline chart; protractor.

Procedure

Always neutralize the right eye first.

(1)   Use the transverse test and rotation test to determine the type of lens.

(2)   If a sphere, determine the sign and form of the lens.

If a sphero-cylinder, determine the cylindrical surface and the approximate axis direction. Using the rotation test, accurately mark the cylinder axis. If the power found by neutralization (step 3) along the cylinder axis meridian is recorded as the sphere, this will ensure that the prescription is finally recorded in the same form in which the lens has been made.

If a toric lens, accurately mark the 'plus axis' meridian of the lens by the rotation test.

(3) Neutralize the lens as described in previous experiments.

(4) Draw the datum line on the lens.

(5) Place the frame on the protractor (front surface down) with the datum line along the 180 meridian of the protractor. Read the axis direction from the protractor. (You may move the lens horizontally to facilitate this, but ensure that the datum line remains parallel with the 180 meridian of the protractor.)

(6) Subtract the reading obtained in step (5) from 180 to obtain the cylinder axis direction in standard notation.

(7) Repeat for the left eye.

(8) On completion, view the lenses from the front and estimate the general axis direction to ensure that it corresponds with the value obtained in step (6). Do not omit this check.

Record your results as shown below.

Frame No.	R.			L.		
	Sph.	Cyl.	Axis	Sph.	Cyl.	Axis

Experiment 30
PRISMS

Theory

A prism is an optical element with plane polished surfaces inclined to one another.

In ophthalmic work, a plano-prism is an optical element with two plane polished surfaces inclined to each other at a small angle.

Figure 30.1 represents the cross section of such a prism. A is the apex and BC is the base. The base setting is the direction of the line from apex to base.

Angle BAC is the apical angle a°. A ray PO is incident normally on the first face of the prism and passes undeviated through the prism. At the second face it is refracted according to the law of refraction and emerges as ray RQ, making an angle d° with its original direction. If n is the refractive index of the prism and the apical angle is small, not exceeding say 10°, then approximately

$$d = (n-1)a \qquad \ldots (1)$$

A proof of this relationship can be obtained as follows.

Figure 30.2 shows the prism ABC with a larger apical angle. From the diagram it can be seen that ray POR is incident on the second face of the prism at an angle of incidence A°. Ray RQ is deviated D° and makes an angle with the normal to the face ARC of value A° + D°.

The law of refraction gives

$$n \sin A = \sin (A + D) \qquad \ldots (2)$$

If the apical angle of the prism becomes very small (5° or less), sin A has approximately the same value as the angle a expressed in radians,

$$\sin A = a \qquad \ldots (3)$$
$$\text{and } \sin (A + D) = a + d \qquad \ldots (4)$$

82

Substituting equations (3) and (4) in equation (2) gives

$$na = a + d$$
$$na - a = d$$
$$\text{or } (n - 1)\,a = d.$$

In ophthalmic work the angle d is measured in prism dioptres. An eye viewing the point P through the prism will see P apparently displaced to the position P′, and the viewing eye will rotate through the angle d and view the image along the direction P′RQ.

Figure 30.1. Ray PO, incident on the prism at O, is refracted by the prism as ray RQ and is deviated through angle d. An eye looking through the prism at an object point at P will see an image of the object at P′. The object has apparently been displaced from P to P′

Figure 30.2. ABC is a prism of large apical angle a. Incident ray PO, normal to the prism face AB, is undeviated and is incident at the second face of the prism, making an angle of incidence a. The angle of refraction is (a + d) and the ray PO has been deviated by angle d

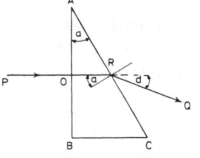

If PP′ is 1 cm and PR is 1 metre, the angle d is defined as $1^\triangle$. An angle of $1^\triangle$ is an angle whose tangent has the value of 0.01; the value of this angle is 34′.

The tangent of 4° is 0.0699 from four-figure tables or $\dfrac{6.99}{100}$. Hence 4° is equivalent to $6.99^\triangle$, and as an approximate working rule, $4° = 7^\triangle$.

83

An angle of $10^\triangle$ is an angle whose tangent is $\dfrac{10}{100}$ or 0.1. This angle is 5°43' or 343'. $1^\triangle$ has the value 34', and 34' × 10 is 340'.

An angle of $100^\triangle$ is an angle whose tangent is $\dfrac{100}{100}$ or 1. This angle is 45° or 2,700'.

$\triangle$	Minutes of angle
1	34
10	343
100	2,700

From the above table it is seen that 100 × $1^\triangle$ has the value of 100 × 34' = 3,400', which is not the value of 2,700', which is $100^\triangle$. This shows that the prism dioptre is not a uniform measure of angle. This is because the tangent of the angle increases at a faster rate than the angle itself. For small angles, however, the discrepancy is small and is neglected in ophthalmic work. This discrepancy is avoided if a unit of deviation equivalent to 0.01 of a radian is used. This unit, termed the centrad, symbol $\triangledown$, is not in general use.

PRISM MEASUREMENT BY TANGENT SCALE

In *Figure 30.1,* if PP' is 4 cm and PO is 2 metres, then d is an angle of $2^\triangle$ (the tangent of the angle is $\dfrac{4}{200}$ or $\dfrac{2}{100}$), hence we would say that the prism has a power of $2^\triangle$. If a scale marked in 2 cm intervals is placed in the plane PP' and PO is 2 metres, the power of the prism can be obtained by direct observation. This is the tangent scale method of determining prism power.

Apparatus

Tangent scale, metre rule, box of prisms of unknown power.

Procedure

(1) Measure the distance between the intervals of the tangent scale. If the distance between the values 0 and 1 is 1 cm, the scale must be

used at 1 metre; if it is 2 cm, the scale must be used at 2 metres. Place the scale horizontally at the correct distance.

(2)   Observe the tangent scale through the unknown prism with one eye (closing the other eye if necessary). Rotate the unknown prism until the base setting is 90°. In this particular position the vertical line of the zero division of the tangent scale will be seen unbroken through and outside the prism.

(3)   Rotate the prism through 90° so that the base setting is horizontal. This can be checked, since in this position the horizontal line of the tangent scale is seen unbroken through and outside the prism. The zero of the tangent scale will be displaced; if the apex of the prism is towards the right, the zero of the scale will be deviated towards the right. When one observes an object through a prism, it is apparently displaced towards the apex.

(4)   Keep the prism steady. Look slowly upward above the prism so that you can see the actual tangent scale. Observe the position of the displaced zero division as seen through the prism compared with the actual tangent scale. The displaced zero mark will apparently coincide with a division on the tangent scale. This position gives the deviation of the prism in prism dioptres. Record this value and the prism number.

(5)   Convert this angle into degrees and calculate the apical angle of the prism in degrees.

Record your results as follows.

Prism No.	Prism dioptres $\triangle$	Degrees of deviation $d°$	$\dfrac{d}{n-1} = a°$

Experiment 31
CONSTRUCTION OF A TANGENT SCALE

Theory

In this experiment we are to construct three scales with a common zero which are to be used at a fixed distance. Hence the apical angle in degrees, the deviation of the prism in degrees, and the deviation of the prism in prism dioptres can be obtained from a fixed position.

Assuming that the scales are to be used at a distance of 2 metres, the divisions for the separate scales can now be calculated.

(1) At 2 metres distance, divisions of 2 cm will subtend an angle whose tangent is $\dfrac{2}{200}$ or 0.01, which is $1^\triangle$. Hence the scale division for prism dioptres will be of magnitude 2 cm.

(2) If at 2 metres a division length x cm subtends $1°$, then $\tan 1° = \dfrac{x}{200}$ and x can be calculated.

To obtain the next division, let $\tan 2° = \dfrac{y}{200}$, hence y can be calculated.

Hence the division for $1°$ is given by $200 \tan 1°$.
"   "   " $2°$ "   "   " $200 \tan 2°$.
"   "   " $3°$ "   "   " $200 \tan 3°$.

Since the angles are small the divisions are virtually equal, hence the magnitude of the scale division for a degree of deviation will be 3.5 cm.

(3) Since $d = (n - 1)a$ for a thin prism,
$$d = 0.523a.$$
$$\text{If } a = 10°, \quad d = 5.23°,$$

hence the scale markings a $= 10°$ and d $= 5.23°$ are of the same magnitude.

Hence the scale marking for $10°$ of apical angle is 5.23×3.5 cm from the zero, therefore the scale marking for $1°$ of apical angle is $\dfrac{5.23 \times 3.5}{10}$ cm from the zero, which is 1.83 cm.

Hence the magnitude of the scale division for $1°$ of apical angle is 1.83 cm. (*See also* Experiment 33.)

Apparatus

Sheet of paper, rule.

Procedure

Two cm from the left edge of the paper, construct a vertical line. This will be the zero for the three scales. Draw three equidistant horizontal lines. Along the top line measure divisions of 2 cm, along the centre line divisions of 3.5 cm, and along the lower line divisions of 1.83 cm. Label the top scale prism dioptres, the centre scale deviation in degrees, and the lower scale apical angle in degrees. Check from your scales that $7^\triangle = 4°$ of deviation and $10°$ apical angle $= 5.23°$ of deviation. The paper should be 37 cm wide to obtain a reading of $10^\triangle$ of prism power. If the sheet of paper is smaller than this, adjust your scales accordingly but mark clearly the distance at which it is to be used.

A model scale is shown in *Figure 31.1.*

Figure 31.1. A model tangent scale. Scale △ reads the power of an unknown prism in prism dioptres. Scale d° reads the power in degrees of deviation. Scale a° reads the apical angle of the prism in degrees for a given refractive index; in this case 1.523. Note: 4° d ≡ 7△ and 5.23° d ≡ 10°a

Experiment 32
DETERMINATION OF REFRACTIVE INDICES OF LIQUIDS USING A CONVEX LENS AND PLANE MIRROR

Theory

This is an extension of the experiment using a plane mirror to determine the focal length of a lens by auto-collimation methods.

Apparatus

Biconvex lens, plane mirror, clamp and pins, spherometer (or lens measure).

Procedure

Place the convex lens on the plane mirror. Hold a pin in a clamp vertically above the mirror and vary the position of the pin until the aerial image of the pin is coincident with the pin. Check the position by parallax and thus obtain the focal length of the lens. Repeat three times and obtain a mean measurement of the focal length and hence the focal power of the lens.

Pour water on the mirror and place the lens on the water, noting which surface of the lens is in contact with the water. The optical system now comprises a convex glass lens and a concave water lens. Determine the focal length of the composite glass water lens, keeping your observations to the central area of the lens where the water is in contact with lens and mirror, and hence the focal power of the system *(Figure 32.1)*.

Determine the radius of curvature of the convex surface of the lens which was in contact with the water, using a spherometer or a lens measure if the lens is made of spectacle crown glass.

DETERMINATION OF REFRACTIVE INDICES OF LIQUIDS

The refractive index of water can now be calculated as follows:

Let F_1 = focal power in dioptres of the convex lens.

F = focal power in dioptres of the convex lens and water lens.

F_w = focal power in dioptres of the water lens.

Then $F = F_1 + F_w$ if the lenses are assumed thin, or

$F - F_1 = F_w$.

Since F and F_1 have been determined experimentally, F_w can be calculated.

Now $F_w = 100 \dfrac{(n_w - 1)}{r}$

where n_w is the refractive index of water and r is the radius of the convex surface in centimetres of the lens in contact with water. Hence n_w can be determined.

Glass
Water

Figure 32.1. Glass lens has focal power F_1; water lens has focal power F_w; total focal power F of the combination is $F_1 + F_w$. The water lens is bounded by the plane surface of the mirror and the curved surface, radius r, of the lens

Clean the mirror and lens and use paraffin as the liquid lens. Determine the focal length of the paraffin and glass lens. Hence determine the refractive index of paraffin.

Exercises

(1) How could you quickly check whether the lens was equiconvex?

(2) In an experiment as above, the focal power of the convex lens was found to be + 9 D. The focal power of the glass water lens was found to be + 6 D. If the radius of curvature of the second surface of the convex lens (in contact with the water) is −11.11 cm, calculate the refractive index of water. (*Answer:* n = 4/3.)

Experiment 33
PRISM MEASUREMENT BY THE ORTHOPS SCALE

Theory

This experiment is to show the relationship between the prism dioptre, the prism dioptre expressed in degrees, and the apical angle of a prism.

The orthops scale consists of a single scale with markings 3.5 cm apart.

(1) If the scale is placed at a distance of 3.5 metres, each division will subtend an angle whose tangent is $\dfrac{3.5}{350}$ or 0.01, hence each division represents $1^{\wedge}$.

(2) To measure directly the deviation of the prism in degrees, let the scale be placed at a distance of x metres or 100x centimetres. Then if each division of the scale is to represent $1°$,

$$\tan 1° = \frac{3.5}{100x}$$

$$0.0175 = \frac{3.5}{100x}$$

$$1.75x = 3.5$$
$$x = 2 \text{ metres.}$$

(3) To measure directly the apical angle $a°$ of the prism assuming that it is made of spectacle glass n = 1.523, let the scale be placed at a distance of z metres. Now d = (n − 1)a. If a is $1°$, then d is $0.523°$. *Figure 33.1* shows a right-angled triangle with one of the angles $0.523°$. If one side is 3.5 cm and the base is of length z metres, then

$$\tan 0.523° = \frac{3.5}{100z} \qquad \qquad \dots (1)$$

90

Hence z can be determined, and each division on the orthops scale will then represent a degree of apical angle.

$$0.523° = 31.38'$$
$$\tan 31.38' = 0.0091 \qquad \ldots(2)$$

Hence from equations (1) and (2),

$$0.0091 = \frac{3.5}{100z}$$

$$z = \frac{3.5}{0.91}$$

$$z = 3.85 \text{ metres.}$$

Therefore if the orthops scale is used at a distance of 3.5 metres, each 3.5 cm division represents $1^\wedge$; if the orthops scale is now placed at a distance of 2 metres, each 3.5 cm division represents $1°$ of deviation; and if the orthops scale is finally used at a distance of 3.85 metres, each 3.5 cm division represents $1°$ apical angle of the prism.

$$\text{Tan } 0.523 = \frac{3.5}{100z}$$

Figure 33.1

Apparatus

Orthops scale, metre rule, prisms.

Procedure

(1) Place the orthops scale in position and measure the distances 3.85, 3.5 and 2 metres from it.

(2) At 3.85 metres from the scale, observe the zero position of the scale through the prism with the base direction of the prism vertical. The procedure is now the same as in steps (2), (3) and (4) of Experiment 30. The prism is rotated $90°$ so that the base direction is horizontal, and the number of divisions by which the zero mark of the orthops scale is apparently displaced is observed. This result gives the apical angle of the prism in degrees.

(3) Now move towards the scale so that you are 3.5 metres from

it. Repeat the precedure in step (2). The number of divisions by which the zero is apparently displaced will give the power of the prism in prism dioptres.

(4)   At 2 metres from the scale, repeat the procedure in step (2). The number of divisions by which the zero is apparently displaced will give the deviation of the prism in degrees.

Record your results as follows.

Prism No.	Apical angle degrees	Prism dioptres △	Degrees deviation

Experiment 34
DETERMINATION OF THE REFRACTIVE INDEX OF A LIQUID

Theory

If a spot is placed on the lower surface of a glass block and an observer looks through the upper surface, the dot appears nearer to the observer. The following experiment is based upon this observation.

Apparatus

Wide tall glass graduated jar; piece of plane mirror to rest across the top of the jar; small pin; large pin; clamp and stand; metre rule.

Procedure

Place a small pin B on the bottom of the cylindrical vessel and put some water in the vessel. Place a strip of plane mirror across the top of the vessel and adjust the position of another pin P until the image of P in the mirror coincides with B', the apparent position of B when viewed from a position vertically above B. Repeat this for various depths l of water. Plot c, the height of the pin above the mirror, as ordinate against l, the depth of water, as abscissa. Find the slope of the graph.

It can be shown that the slope of the graph has the value $\dfrac{1-n}{n}$.

From this determine the refractive index of water.

Notes on the graph

The proof of the experiment is as follows.

Figure 34.1 illustrates the jar of depth b containing a liquid of refractive index n and depth l. Pin B is imaged at B' at the apparent depth l' below the surface of the liquid. B′ is located by the distance c, which represents the position of pin P above the mirror when there is no parallax between pin P and the image B′ of pin B.

Figure 34.1

It was shown in Experiment 14 that $l' = \dfrac{l}{n}$.

$$\text{Since } c = l' + b - l$$

$$= \frac{l}{n} - l + b$$

$$\text{we find } c \; = \; \left(\frac{1-n}{n} \right) l + b,$$

so that when c is plotted vertically against l, the slope of the straight line which is obtained is $\dfrac{1-n}{n}$.

Experiment 35
NEUTRALIZATION OF PRISMS

Theory

When an object is viewed through a prism it is apparently displaced towards the apex or thin edge of the prism. Take a $10^\triangle$ prism from the neutralizing set and view a crossline chart through it. That part of the crossline chart viewed through the prism will be displaced and the crosslines will appear broken. Move the prism laterally and observe that there is no change in the appearance of the crosslines. Hence when the transverse test is applied to a prism there is no such 'with' or 'against' movement as one obtains when the test is applied to a lens. Thus the transverse test distinguishes between a lens and a plano prism.

Rotate the prism in its own plane and note that the crosslines rotate with it. Place a $6^\triangle$ prism in contact with the $10^\triangle$ prism, base to apex, so that the total power of the composite prism is $4^\triangle$. Again rotate the composite prism. It will be observed that the apparent rotation of the crosslines is less. This is the basis of a method for determining the power of unknown prisms by neutralization. The method is more sensitive if the crossline chart is viewed at a distance.

Apparatus

Neutralizing set; crossline chart; box of unknown prisms.

Procedure

(1) Mark the base setting of the unknown prism.

(2) View the crossline chart through the prism and estimate the power of the prism.

(3) Take a prism of this power from the neutralizing set and place it in contact, base to apex, with the unknown prism.

(4) View the crosslines through the composite prism and note their apparent displacement. Apply the rotation test. The crosslines will be displaced towards the apex of the composite prism. Modify the neutralizing prism until the rotation test shows no movement of the crosslines. When this occurs, the neutralizing prism is the power in prism dioptres of the unknown prism.

(5) Record your results.

Experiment 36
DETERMINATION OF REFRACTIVE INDEX BY MEASUREMENT OF THE BREWSTER ANGLE

Theory

Obtain two pieces of Polaroid sheet. Pass a beam of light through either piece, and the transmitted beam apparently does not differ (apart from absorption effects) from the incident beam.

Place the two pieces together. Rotate one sheet with respect to the other. It will be found that the transmitted beam gradually fades until a position is reached where the light is completely extinguished. A further rotation of $90°$ restores the original transmission of the beam.

It would appear that the light, after passing through the Polaroid first sheet, has been modified so that it is only transmitted by the second sheet when this is in a certain position.

Each Polaroid sheet has a direction known as the optic axis. If the two sheets are placed together with their optic axes parallel, the beam of light is transmitted. If one sheet is now rotated $90°$ so that the optic axes are perpendicular to each other, no light is transmitted.

It would appear that the light, after passing through the Polaroid sheet, has acquired a property of transmission in one plane. The particular nature of this need not concern us here. This light is said to be plane polarized and will only be transmitted for a particular position of the second Polaroid sheet.

When a beam of ordinary light is incident on a surface separating two media, the reflected light can be considered to be a mixture of ordinary and plane polarized light. At a certain angle of incidence, all the reflected light is plane polarized. This angle, known as the Brewster angle ϕ_B, is given by $\tan \phi_B = n$ where n is the refractive index of the medium bounded by the reflecting surface.

The object of this experiment is to find ϕ_B for various materials and liquids, and thus to determine their refractive indices.

97

Apparatus

Material or liquid under test; point source of light (filament lamps); sheet of Polaroid P.

Procedure

Set up the apparatus as shown in *Figure 36.1*.
Rotate the polarizer to give a minimum intensity of light reflected

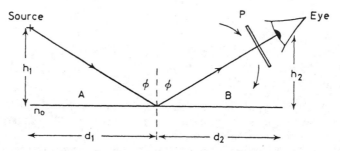

Figure 36.1. Source is at height h_1 above surface bounding media refractive index n_0 and air. Ray of light from source is reflected by surface into eye. P represents a polarizing filter before source and eye; h_2 is the height of the observing eye above the surface. If the light entering the eye is plane polarized, ϕ is the Brewster angle and
$$\tan \phi = n_0$$

from the surface AB. Vary the height of the eye until a position for minimum intensity is found. Make these adjustments alternately. Measure the distances indicated in *Figure 36.1*.

Then $n_0 = \tan \phi_B = \dfrac{d_1}{h_1} = \dfrac{d_2}{h_2}$

and hence n_0 may be determined.

Carry out the experiment for both liquid and glass surfaces. Keep h_1 constant and take about ten readings for d_1.

Experiment 37
EDGE THICKNESS DIFFERENCE OF
A PRISM

Theory

The thinnest and thickest edges of a plano-prism are the apex and base edges respectively. The base setting is the direction of the line from apex to base in a principal section. The principal section lies in a plane perpendicular to the refracting edge of the prism.

Figure 37.1. Plano-prism. AD = refracting edge or apex of prism; BCFE = base of prism; ADFC and ADEB = refracting faces; ABC and DEF = principal sections

In *Figure 37.1*, AD is the refracting edge. ABC is a principal section of the plano-prism. Angle BAC is the apical angle of the prism. BC is the base, the thickest part of the principal section. At A the apex is knife-edged or zero thickness. The apex is the intersection of the refracting edge AD with a principal section. DEF is another principal section of the prism.

If BC = the prism thickness difference, g, and AB = the diameter of the plano-prism, b, and we denote the refractive index of the prism by n and the power of the prism in dioptres by P, then, assuming that the apex is knife-edged,

$$P = \frac{100 \, g \, (n - 1)}{b}$$

99

This equation can be derived from *Figure 30.1* (*see* Experiment 30). In *Figure 30.1*, ABC represents the end face of the prism under consideration.

BC = g, since there is zero thickness at A.

Tan a $= \dfrac{g}{b}$ and by definition 100 tan a = the apical angle, a, expressed in prism dioptres.

Hence a, in prism dioptres, $= \dfrac{100\,g}{b}$ ...(1)

Now it was shown in Experiment 30 that

$$d = (n - 1)\,a$$

where d is the deviation produced by a prism of small apical angle, a, and n is the refractive index.

If a is expressed in prism dioptres, d will be given in prism dioptres. The deviation produced by a prism in dioptres is the power of the prism P, so we can write

$$P = (n - 1)\,a \qquad \qquad ...(2)$$
(P and a in prism dioptres)

Hence, combining equations (1) and (2),

$$P = \frac{100\,g\,(n - 1)}{b} \qquad \qquad ...(3)$$

Rearranging equation (3), we find

$$g = \frac{P.b}{100\,(n - 1)} \qquad \qquad ...(4)$$

Equation (4) provides solutions which are accurate only for prisms of small apical angle.

An exact relationship can be derived from *Figure 30.2*. It was shown in the text accompanying this illustration that

$$n \sin a = \sin (a + d).$$

Expanding this equation, we find

$$n \sin a = \sin a \cos d + \cos a \sin d,$$

or $\sin a\,(n - \cos d) = \cos a \sin d.$

$$\therefore \frac{\sin a}{\cos a} = \frac{\sin d}{n - \cos d}$$

$$\text{or } \tan a = \frac{\sin d}{n - \cos d} \qquad \dots (5)$$

$$\text{Since } \tan a = \frac{BC}{AB} = \frac{g}{b}$$

$$\text{we have } g = \frac{b. \sin d}{n - \cos d} \qquad \dots (6)$$

When angle d is small, as in most ophthalmic prisms, $\sin d \to \tan d$ and $\cos d \to 1$, and so

$$g = \frac{b \tan d}{n - 1}$$

Since $P = 100 \tan d$, $g = \dfrac{b.P}{100 (n - 1)}$, which is equation (4).

Apparatus

Lens thickness calipers; crossline chart; set of prisms with at least one prism of high power, say $10^\triangle$.

Procedure

(1) Mark the base setting of the prism.

(2) Measure along this direction a convenient distance, 40 or 50 mm or, if possible, 52.3 mm, and mark two points this distance apart. This is the distance b in equation (3).

(3) Measure the thickness of the prism at these two points with the thickness calipers and subtract the lesser reading from the greater to obtain the thickness difference g.

(4) Use equation (3) to calculate the power of the prism under test. The result is given in prism dioptres.

If b = 52.3 mm, the numerical work is considerably reduced, for from equation (3), substituting 1.523 for n,

$$P = \frac{100 \, g \, (0.523)}{52.3}$$

or P = g.

That is, the thickness difference g in millimetres gives numerically the power of the prism in dioptres.

Record your results as follows.

Prism No.	Thickness 1	Thickness 2	$[= 1\overset{g}{-} 2]$	$\left[= \dfrac{100\,g\,(n-1)}{b}\right]$

(5)   A result for the high-powered prism ($10^\triangle$ or so) will have been obtained using equation (3). For this prism, use the following method to obtain a more accurate value for P.

Tan $a = \dfrac{g}{b}$. Hence find angle a.

Use $n \sin a = \sin (a + d)$ to find angle d.
Use $P = 100 \tan d$ to find P.

Compare the results of this sequence with those obtained from equation (3). Are you justified in concluding that, in general, equation (3) is sufficiently accurate?

Exercise

Show that the thickness difference g for a prism of power $P^\triangle$ and diameter b is given by the exact relationship

$$g = \frac{\dfrac{b.P}{100}}{n\left(\sqrt{\left[1 + \left(\dfrac{P}{100}\right)^2\right]}\right) - 1}$$

Experiment 38
DISPERSIVE POWER OF A LENS:
TELESCOPE METHOD

Theory

When an object is placed at one of the principal foci of a positive lens, the light proceeding from each point of it is rendered parallel on emergence from the lens and so will be sharply focused by a telescope adjusted for infinity.

If, therefore, a telescope is focused on a very distant object or on a collimator and placed in position following the lens, the object will be distinctly seen only when it is placed at the principal focus of the lens. If the powers, F_F', F_d and F_C' of the lens for blue, yellow and red light respectively are found, the dispersive power can be calculated by substituting in the formal

$$\omega = \frac{F_F' - F_C'}{F_d}$$

Apparatus

Optical bench; astronomical telescope; lenses to be tested; object; blue, yellow and red filters.

Procedure

Focus the telescope for parallel light, using a very distant object and a filter. On optical bench set up lamp, filter, object, lens and telescope in that order. Move the object until it is clearly seen through the lens and telescope. The object is then at the principal focus of the lens and their separation is the focal length of the lens (strictly this separation is the focusing distance or vertex focal length of the lens). Record positions of object and lens.

Repeat three times and obtain the mean value. Repeat for all the lenses provided. Use the filters in the order blue, yellow, red.

Tabulate your results as follows.

103

Lens No.	Position of		Focal length f' (cm)			Power of lens $F = \dfrac{100}{f'}$ (dioptres)			Dispersive power ω $= \dfrac{F_F' \, F_C'}{F_d}$
	Object	Lens	Blue	Yellow	Red	Blue	Yellow	Red	

Conclusions

Of what type of glass is the lens probably made? Is this method reliable?

Exercises

(1) Show by a clear diagram how you would use the telescope method to determine the focal length of a negative lens.

(2) If an object 1 cm high is placed at the principal focus of a positive lens of focal length 20 cm and observed with a telescope adjusted for infinity as in the experiment, what will be the size of the image formed at the principal focus of the telescope objective if the focal length of this objective is 40 cm? Draw a diagram. (*Answer:* 2 cm.)

(3) Derive the formula given above for dispersive power, ω, where

$$\omega = \frac{n_{F'} - n_{C'}}{n_d - 1}$$

Hint. – Use $F_{F'} = (n_{F'} - 1) R$, etc., and substitute.

Experiment 39
MARKING AND SETTING PLANO-PRISMS

Theory

Objects viewed through a prism appear displaced towards the prism apex. Thus the limbs of a crossline chart viewed through a plano-prism will appear displaced towards the prism apex, the displacement depending upon the position of the prism in relation to the chart. Suppose that a plano-prism is held before a crossline chart with its base setting (or base—apex direction) parallel to the vertical limb of the chart. Only the horizontal crossline will appear to be displaced as shown in *Figure 39.1a.*

If the prism is rotated clockwise, the crosslines also appear to rotate but remain at right angles to each other, always being displaced towards the prism apex *(Figure 39.1b).* If the rotation is continued until the base setting is horizontal, only the vertical line will appear to be broken *(Figure 39.1c).*

When the prism is rotated into the position shown in *Figure 39.1a,* the base setting can be marked. Two short lines at the extremities of the base—apex direction represent the base setting, and a short horizontal line represents the base edge of the prism *(Figure 39.2).*

When the base setting has been marked, the prism may be set to an individual prescription.

The base setting may lie in any direction, and the following notation is used to describe the direction.

Each eye is divided into two halves, UP and DOWN, and the standard cylinder axis notation is used to determine the base setting. If the base setting is to be UP, DOWN, IN (towards the nose) or OUT (towards the temple), there is no need to specify an axis direction; the prism power is written accompanied by one of these four instructions.

When the base setting is oblique, however, the position of the base is indicated by stating whether it lies above or below the horizontal meridian and also its particular axis direction.

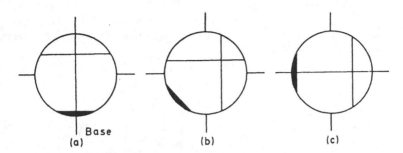

Base
(a)   (b)   (c)

Figure 39.1. Objects viewed through a prism appear to be displaced towards the prism apex. Thus, when a prism is held base down before a crossline chart the horizontal limb of the chart appears to be displaced upwards (a). Rotation of the prism in a clockwise direction produces the successive appearances shown in (b) and (c)

Thus the base setting shown in *Figure 39.4* would be written as follows.

(1) P△ base UP at 60.
(2) P△ base DOWN at 120.

The object of this experiment is to mark and set assorted plano-prisms to individual prescriptions ready for the glazing process. The base setting is found first and then the prism is marked for glazing as described in Experiment 23.

Figure 39.2. Marking the base setting for a plano-prism. The short horizontal line represents the base edge of the prism

Apparatus

Box of plano-prisms together with written instructions for the base setting of each; centring machine; protractor; tangent scale (to determine the power of each prism); waterproof ink and brush or pen or grease pencil (for practice use).

107

Procedure

(1) Sort out the prisms by means of the tangent scale to match the individual instruction forms.

(2) Hold the prism before the crossline chart and rotate until the vertical limb of the chart is continuous both within and outside the prism. The base setting now lies in the vertical meridian and can be marked as shown in *Figure 39.2.*

Figure 39.3. Standard notation for base setting. Each eye is divided into two halves, UP and DOWN. Standard axis notation is used for oblique base settings. N is the nasal side of each eye

(3) Place the prism on the protractor with its mid-point at the intersection of the 90 and 180 meridians of the protractor and rotate the prism so that the base setting lies along the prescribed meridian. (If the prism is curved in form, make sure that the front surface lies uppermost.)

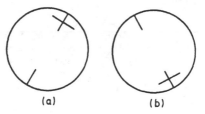

Figure 39.4. (a) R. base setting is UP at 60. (b) L. base setting is DOWN at 120

(4) Using waterproof ink, draw a thin straight cutting line along the horizontal meridian of the prism, following the 180 meridian of the protractor. This line should pass through the mid-point of the prism.

(5) Draw a shorter vertical line along the vertical meridian of the prism, following the 90 meridian of the protractor.

(6) Indicate which eye the prism is to be used before by marking R or L in the upper temporal quadrant of the prism and by drawing an arrowhead near the nasal end of the horizontal cutting line as shown in *Figure 23.1.*

Experiment 40
COMPOUNDING PRISM POWERS

Theory

When a prescription calls for two prismatic powers to be combined in one lens, the prisms may be compounded together into a single prismatic effect. Thus a prescription may call for a lens to include $3^\triangle$ base UP and $4^\triangle$ base IN. These effects can be achieved by using a single prism of power $5^\triangle$ placed with its base setting UP along $37°$ (assuming the prism is to be used for the right eye). This process of adding together two prisms inclined at an angle to each other is known as *compounding* prism powers.

The procedure for compounding prisms is quite straightforward and may be performed by a simple graphical construction or by calculation. The methods will be explained by means of the following examples.

Examples

(1)   Compound $3^\triangle$ base UP and $4^\triangle$ base IN into a single prismatic effect for the right eye.

The graphical solution is shown in *Figure 40.1*. The rules for the construction are as follows.

(a)   Construct 90 and 180 meridians and indicate the nasal side.
(b)   Choosing a suitable scale, say 1 cm represents $1^\triangle$, construct two lines representing $3^\triangle$ base UP and $4^\triangle$ base IN (OV and OH in *Figure 40.1*).
(c)   Complete the rectangle OVRH and draw the diagonal OR. The length of OR represents the magnitude of the resultant prism, and angle ROH gives its direction in standard notation.

From *Figure 40.1* we find OR = $5^\triangle$ and angle ROH = $37°$.
Therefore right eye $3^\triangle$ UP $\circeq$ $4^\triangle$ IN $\equiv$ $5^\triangle$ UP at $37°$.

110

This result could also have been obtained as follows.

By Pythagoras' theorem, $OR = \sqrt{(OV^2 + OH^2)}$
$$= \sqrt{(3^2 + 4^2)}$$
$$= \sqrt{25}$$
$$= 5$$

and $\tan ROH = \dfrac{OV}{OH} = \dfrac{3}{4} = 0.75$

$\therefore$ angle $ROH = \tan^{-1} 0.75 = 36° 52'$.

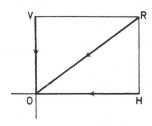

Figure 40.1. Compounding prism powers. Length OV is 3 units long and represents $3^\triangle$ base UP. It is drawn in an upward direction from the origin O. Length OH is 4 units long and represents $4^\triangle$ base IN (for the right eye). Completing the parallelogram OHRV and drawing the diagonal OR enables the single resultant prism, represented by length OR, to be found. By measurement OR = 5 units and $\measuredangle$ ROH = 37°. Hence $3^\triangle$ base UP $\circ$ $4^\triangle$ base IN $\equiv$ $5^\triangle$ base UP at 37°

(2) Compound $1^\triangle$ base **DOWN** and $2^\triangle$ base IN into a single prismatic effect for the right eye.

The graphical construction is shown in *Figure 40.2*.

By measurement, OR = $2.24^\triangle$ base **DOWN** at 153½°.

By Pythagoras' theorem, $OR = \sqrt{(1^2 + 2^2)}$
$$= 2.24^\triangle$$

Tan ROH = ½ = 0.5, and angle ROH = 26°34'.
In standard notation the final base setting is $180 - ROH = 153°26'$.
$\therefore$ resultant = $2.24^\triangle$ base DOWN at 153° 26'.

In the following experiment, two prisms of known strength are placed together with their base settings at right angles to each other and their resultant effect is determined by means of a tangent scale. Also the base setting of the resultant effect can be marked and the direction of the resultant effect found by means of a protractor.

Apparatus

Box of plano-prisms; tangent scale; protractor; grease pencil; cross-line chart.

Procedure

(1) Using the crossline chart, mark the base setting of each prism as described in Experiment 39.

(2) By means of the tangent scale, determine the power of each prism.

(3) Place the two prisms together with their base settings at right

Figure 40.2. Draw OV, 1 unit in length, to represent $1^\triangle$ base DOWN. Draw OH, 2 units in length, to represent $2^\triangle$ IN. Complete the parallelogram OVRH and draw the diagonal OR. By measurement, OR = 2.24 units and ⦝ VOR = 63½°. In standard notation, the resultant prism is $2.24^\triangle$ base DOWN at 153½°. In practice this would be made as a $2.25^\triangle$ prism base DOWN at 153½°

angles to each other and, using the crossline chart, mark the base setting of the new single prismatic effect. Make sure that you do not rotate either prism.

(4) Keeping the prisms firmly in contact, hold the pair before the tangent scale and determine the new resultant power of the combination.

(5) Place the prisms on a protractor with their base settings along the 90 and 180 meridians of the protractor and record the angle between the prism whose base setting lies along 180 and the new base setting of the combination.

(6) Check your results by calculation as shown in the following table.

112

Prism 1 (vertical)	Prism 2 (horizontal)	Resultant prism	Base setting	$P_1{}^2$	$P_2{}^2$
$2^\triangle$ UP	$3^\triangle$ IN	$3.6^\triangle$	UP at 33½°	4	9
$P_1{}^2 + P_2{}^2$	OR	$\tan ROH$	ROH		
	$\sqrt{(P_1{}^2 + P_2{}^2)}$	$\dfrac{P_1}{P_2}$		Resultant prism	
13	3.61	0.6667	33°42'	3.61$^\triangle$ base UP at 33° 42'	

Experiment 41
THE PRISMATIC EFFECT OF A THIN
LENS

Theory

A ray of light will be deviated by a lens unless it passes through the optical centre.

Figure 41.1 shows a thin biconvex lens; C_1 C_2 is the optical axis. All rays such as AB parallel to the axis pass through the second focal point F'. Rays at appreciable distances from the optical centre pass almost through F', cutting the optical axis nearer to the lens from F'. This effect is known as spherical aberration and will be neglected in this elementary treatment.

Ray DE is incident on the lens at a greater distance from the optical axis than AB and is deviated through an angle θ_2; ray AB is deviated through angle θ_1, and $\theta_2 > \theta_1$.

In ophthalmic prescription work, angles θ_1 and θ_2 are measured in prism dioptres. A prism dioptre is an angle whose tangent is 1/100. This statement is sometimes written as

$$\tan^{-1} \left(\frac{1}{100} \right) = 1 \text{ prism dioptre}$$
$$= 1^{\triangle}.$$

In the right-angled triangle ABC *(Figure 41.2)*, if AB is 1 unit and BC is 100 units, then tan ACB is 1/100 and angle ACB, denoted by θ, is $1^{\triangle}$.

Hence $\tan \theta = 1/100$ ...(1)
   and $\theta = 1^{\triangle}$.

Figure 41.1. Rays AB and DE, parallel to the optical axis C_2OC_1, are deviated through angles θ_2 and θ_1 respectively. Ray C_2O passes undeviated through the lens. O is the optical centre of the lens. Distance OB is the decentration of ray AB. Distance OE is the decentration of ray DE. Angle θ_1 in prism dioptres is given by OB x F where OB is expressed in centimetres and F is the focal power of the lens

Figure 41.2

In *Figure 41.1*, ray AB is distant c centimetres from the optical axis.

Then $\tan \theta_1 = \dfrac{c \text{ cm}}{f' \text{ cm}}$ ...(2)

If the focal power of the lens is F dioptres, then by definition,

$$F = \frac{1}{f' \text{ metres}} = \frac{100}{f' \text{ cm}}$$ ...(3)

Combining equations (2) and (3),

$$\tan \theta_1 = \frac{cF}{100}$$ ...(4)

Combining equations (1) and (4),

$$\theta_1 = cF \text{ prism dioptres.}$$

θ_1 is termed the prismatic effect of the lens at the point B and is expressed in prism dioptres, denoted by the symbol P. Note that c must be expressed in centimetres and F in dioptres.

Hence $P = cF$.

Apparatus

Drawing board; paper and pins; rule; small transparent scale; 'bisected' ophthalmic lens with lens holders; ray box; protractor.

Procedure

(1) (a) Determine the optical centre of the lens. This is the position through which an incident ray is undeviated. Set the half lens in the holders so that the straight edge is in contact with the paper. Place the ray box on the paper and arrange for only one ray of light to emerge from the ray box. From this determine the optical centre. Note that if

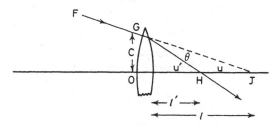

Figure 41.3. Ray FG is not parallel to the axis and is deviated through angle θ. Angle θ in prism dioptres is given by OG x F where OG is expressed in centimetres and F is the focal power of the lens

Figure 41.4

the ray is incident on any other portion of the lens, it will be deviated. Mark the position of the optical centre on the paper and draw the optical axis. Note that this must be normal to both surfaces of the lens.

(b) Arrange that a ray from the ray box is incident on the lens, parallel to the optical axis and distant c cm from it. The refracted ray

116

will be deviated. Measure this angle of deviation θ. Obtain values of θ for various values of c (c could be 4, 8, 12, 16 or 20 mm). Plot a graph of 100 tan θ against c cm (*see Figure 41.4*).

(c) Determine the value of the slope of the graph. What does it represent? Record this value and the number engraved on the lens.

So far we have considered rays parallel to the axis. We must now consider the general case where the rays are not parallel to the optical axis.

Figure 41.3 shows ray FG deviated through angle θ after refraction.

From the geometry of *Figure 41.3*,

$$u' = u + \theta.$$

Hence $\theta = u' - u$.

Now u' in prism dioptres $= \dfrac{OG \times 100}{l'}$.

and u in prism dioptres $= \dfrac{OG \times 100}{l}$

$\therefore \theta$ in prism dioptres $= 100 \times OG \left(\dfrac{1}{l'} - \dfrac{1}{l}\right).$

Calling OG c and expressing this distance in centimetres,

$$\theta = c \left(\frac{1}{l'} - \frac{1}{l}\right) \text{prism dioptres.}$$

The term in parentheses will be recognized as the lens power F (*see* Experiment 17). Hence $\theta = cF$.

(2) Repeat as for (1), arranging that the rays from the ray box are incident on the lens but are not parallel to the optical axis. Obtain values of θ (*see Figure 41.3*) for various values of c and plot a graph of 100 tan θ against c (*Figure 41.4*).

Exercises

(1) Show how your result could have been obtained by a direct measurement.

(a) A ray parallel to and distant 8 mm from the optical axis is incident on a thin lens of power + 4 D. What is the deviation of the refracted ray in prism dioptres?

(b) Repeat as for (a) with the ray inclined at an angle of 10° with the optical axis.

Experiment 42
THE PRISMATIC EFFECT AT ANY
POINT ON A LENS

Theory

It is often necessary to calculate the prismatic effect introduced when the eye looks through various points of a lens. When the lens is spherical, the prismatic effect can usually be calculated mentally, but when the lens incorporates a cylindrical component the procedure is a little more complicated.

Spherical lenses

If we assume that a spherical lens is mounted before an eye with the optical centre of the lens directly in front of the eye's pupil, then the base direction of the prismatic effect which is exerted by the lens can be easily determined from a simple sketch such as *Figure 42.1*.

Figure 42.1a shows a positive spherical lens which is supposed to be mounted before the right eye. The cross-sectional views of the lens show immediately the effect of the lens in the vertical and horizontal meridians. Thus if the eye were to look through the point a, the prismatic effect at a would be clearly base DOWN. If the eye looks through the point b, the prismatic effects which are encountered can be seen to be base UP and base OUT, which effects may be compounded into a single effect base UP and OUT.

Figure 42.1b shows a spherical negative lens which is supposed to be mounted before the left eye. From the cross-sectional views of the lens we can see that the prismatic effect at point a is base UP, whereas the prismatic effect at point b is base DOWN and base IN.

The magnitude of these prismatic effects is calculated from the expression derived in Experiment 41, where $P = cF$. P is the prismatic

118

effect in prism dioptres, c is the distance of the point in question from the optical centre of the lens measured in centimetres, and F is the lens power in dioptres (D).

Figure 42.1. (a) Plus lens, right eye. OC is the optical centre of the lens and represents the position of the prism base for any point on the lens. Thus at point a which lies above OC, the prismatic effect is base DOWN. At point b, OC lies up and out and the prismatic effect is also base UP and OUT. (b) Minus lens left eye. OC is the optical centre of the lens and represents the position of the prism apex for any point on the lens. Thus at point a the prismatic effect has its apex below a and its base above a, i.e., the prismatic effect at a is base UP. The prismatic effect at point b is base DOWN and IN

Thus if the lens shown in *Figure 42.1a* is a + 4.00 DS (right eye) and the point a lies 9 mm above the optical centre, then

$$P = cF$$
$$= 0.9 \times 4$$
$$= 3.6^\triangle \text{ base DOWN.}$$

The prismatic effect at the point b, which lies 8 mm below and 5 mm inwards from the optical centre, would be:

Vertically $\quad P_V = c_V F$
$$= 0.8 \times 4$$
$$= 3.2^\triangle \text{ base UP.}$$

Horizontally, $P_H = c_H F$
$$= 0.5 \times 4$$
$$= 2^\triangle \text{ base OUT.}$$

These vertical and horizontal prismatic effects may be compounded into a single resultant effect using the methods of Experiment 40.

119

The resultant effect, P_R, $= \sqrt{(P_V^2 + P_H^2)}$
$$= \sqrt{(3.2^2 + 2^2)}$$
$$= \sqrt{(14.24)}$$
$$\therefore P_R = 3.77^\triangle$$

The direction of this effect in standard notation is

$$180 - \tan^{-1} \frac{P_V}{P_H} = 180 - \tan^{-1} 1.6$$

$$= (180 - 58) \text{ or } 122^\circ$$

$$\therefore P_R = 3.77^\triangle \text{ base UP at } 122.$$

Cylindrical lenses

There is no power along the axis meridian of a cylinder and so there can be no prismatic effect exerted along this meridian. The power of a

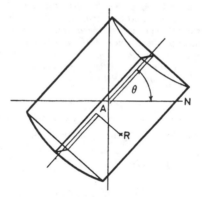

Figure 42.2. The prismatic effect at point R is the product of the perpendicular distance of R from the cylinder axis, AR, measured in centimetres, and the power of the cylinder in dioptres. The prismatic effect lies along the direction AR, or 90 + θ

cylinder lies at right angles to its axis meridian, and hence a cylinder exerts prismatic effect only along its power meridian at right angles to its axis.

Figure 42.2 shows a plano-convex cylinder with its axis inclined at an angle θ to the horizontal meridian. Assume that it is mounted before

120

the right eye. The prismatic effect at the point R is simply the product of the perpendicular distance of the point R from the cylinder axis in centimetres (AR) and the power of the cylinder. The diagram shows that the prism base must lie UP and OUT for the right eye.

If we require the vertical and horizontal prismatic effects only, we could resolve the distance AR into vertical and horizontal components and multiply these by the power of the cylinder. The procedure is shown diagrammatically in *Figure 42.3*. The cylinder is represented

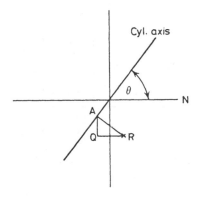

Figure 42.3. The vertical and horizontal prismatic effects at R can be found by resolving the distance AR into vertical and horizontal components, AQ and QR respectively. The product of AQ, in centimetres, and the focal power of the cylinder in dioptres is the vertical prismatic effect at R. The product of QR, in centimetres, and the power of the cylinder is the horizontal prismatic effect at R

only by its axis meridian, drawn along its prescribed direction. To find the prismatic effect at the point R, a perpendicular is dropped from R to the cylinder axis, meeting it at A, and AR is resolved into vertical and horizontal components, AQ and QR respectively. Expressing the distances AQ and QR in centimetres, we have only to multiply these by the power of the cylinder to obtain the vertical and horizontal prismatic effects.

The rules for this construction may be summarized as follows.

Procedure

(1)   Construct 90 and 180 meridians of lens indicating nasal side.

(2)   Treating the intersection of 90 and 180 meridians as the geometrical centre of the cylinder (or, if the lens is a sph.-cyl., as the position of the optical centre – *see below*), locate and mark the position of the point R. Choose the largest scale that your paper permits, e.g., let 1 cm represent 1 mm.

(3)   Draw the cylinder axis through the origin along its prescribed direction.

Figure 42.4. By measurement: $AQ = 0.32$ cm and $QR = 0.56$ cm

$$P_V = AQ \times F_{cyl} = 0.32 \times 4 = 1.28^\triangle \text{ base DOWN}$$
$$P_H = QR \times F_{cyl} = 0.56 \times 4 = 2.24^\triangle \text{ base IN}$$

The base directions can be verified from the cross-sectional sketch of the minus cylinder

(4)   Draw a perpendicular from R to the cylinder axis (AR in *Figure 42.3*).

(5)   Resolve AR into vertical and horizontal components (AQ and QR respectively in *Figure 42.3*).

(6)   Measure AQ and express in centimetres. Multiply this by the power of the cylinder to obtain the vertical prismatic effect. Measure QR and express in centimetres. Multiply this by the power of the cylinder to obtain the horizontal prismatic effect.

(7)   Sketch the form of the cylinder to determine the base direction.

Example

Find the prismatic effect at a point 6 mm below and 4 mm inwards from the geometric centre of the cylinder L. -4.00×120.

The construction is shown in *Figure 42.4*.

By measurement, AQ = 0.32 cm and QR = 0.56 cm.

Vertical prismatic effect P_V = AQ $\times$ F_{cyl} = 0.32 $\times$ 4
$$= 1.28^\triangle.$$

Horizontal prismatic effect P_H = QR $\times$ F_{cyl} = 0.56 $\times$ 4
$$= 2.24^\triangle.$$

Figure 42.4 shows that the base directions must be DOWN and IN, i.e., $P_V = 1.28^\triangle$ base DOWN and $P_H = 2.24^\triangle$ base IN.

Sphero-cylindrical lenses

A sphero-cylindrical lens may be considered as a sphere and a separate cylinder, so by combining the prismatic effects found for the spherical element of a lens with the effects found for the cylindrical element we can find the prismatic effects at any point on an astigmatic lens.

Examples

(1) Find the prismatic effects at a point 6 mm below and 4 mm inwards from the optical centre of the lens. L. $-3.00/-4.00 \times 120$.

Prism due to sphere

$$P_V = c_V F_{sph}$$
$$= 0.6 \times 3$$
$$= 1.8^\triangle \text{ base DOWN}$$

$$\text{and } P_H = c_H F_{sph}$$
$$= 0.4 \times 3$$
$$= 1.2^\triangle \text{ base IN.}$$

Prism due to cylinder

The prismatic effect of the cylindrical element of this lens has been found in the previous example.

We had $P_V = 1.28^\triangle$ base DOWN,
$$P_H = 2.24^\triangle \text{ base IN.}$$

123

Adding the prismatic effect of the sphere we find:

Total P_V = $3.08^\triangle$ base DOWN
      = $3.44^\triangle$ base IN.

(2)   Find the prismatic effect at a point 8 mm above and 3 mm inwards from the optical centre of the lens R. $- 6.00/ + 2.00 \times 40$.

Prism due to sphere

$$P_V = c_V\ F_{sph}$$
$$= 0.8 \times 6$$
$$= 4.8^\triangle\ base\ UP$$

$$and\ P_H = c_H\ F_{sph}$$
$$= 0.3 \times 6$$
$$= 1.8^\triangle\ base\ IN.$$

Figure 42.5. By measurement: AQ = 0.32 cm and QR = 0.27 cm
$$P_V = AQ \times F_{cyl} = 0.32 \times 2 = 0.64^\triangle\ base\ DOWN$$
$$P_H = QR \times F_{cyl} = 0.27 \times 2 = 0.54^\triangle\ base\ IN$$

Prism due to cylinder

The graphical construction is shown in *Figure 42.5.*
By measurement, AQ = 0.32 cm
                    QR = 0.27 cm

$$\therefore P_V = AQ \times F_{cyl}$$
$$= 0.32 \times 2$$
$$= 0.64^\triangle \text{ base DOWN (see } Figure\ 42.5).$$
$$P_H = QR \times F_{cyl}$$
$$= 0.27 \times 2$$
$$= 0.54^\triangle \text{ base IN.}$$

Adding the prism due to the sphere, we have:

$$\text{Total } P_V = 4.16^\triangle \text{ base UP}$$
$$P_H = 2.34^\triangle \text{ base IN.}$$

Experiment 43
MARKING AND SETTING OF SPHERICAL LENSES WHICH INCORPORATE DECENTRATION

Theory

A decentred lens is one whose optical centre does not coincide with its standard optical centre position. The latter is a reference point on each lens at which the optical centre is placed by a prescription house in the absence of prescribed decentration or prismatic effect. It lies on the vertical line which passes through the datum centre of the lens, but its actual height depends upon the particular prescription house.

Spectacle lenses are usually decentred for one of the following two reasons:

(1)   Because the subject's centration point does not coincide with the standard optical centre position of the lens which he is to wear.

(2)   In order to produce a prescribed prismatic effect at the subject's centration point.

Whichever reason necessitates the decentration of a spherical lens, it is essential to ensure that the decentration required can be obtained from the given uncut size. If the uncut lens diameter is large enough to accommodate the finished decentred lens, the decentration can be performed during the marking and setting process.

The following examples should make the procedure clear.

Examples

(1)   Decentre the lens R. + 5.00 DS 3 mm upwards and 2 mm inwards.

When the lens is edged, its optical centre must lie 3 mm above and 2 mm to the nasal side of the standard optical centre position. The

126

cutting lines marked on the lens during the laying-off process intersect at the standard optical centre position. The lens, after laying off, should therefore have the appearance shown in *Figure 43.1a.*

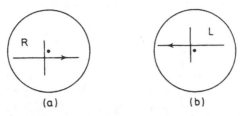

Figure 43.1. The cutting lines intersect at the standard optical centre position. The dots indicate the positions of the optical centres

(2) Decentre the lens L. − 4.00 DS to produce $1^\triangle$ base UP and $1^\triangle$ base IN.

Here the decentration is not stated directly but must first be calculated from the decentration formula $c = \dfrac{P}{F}$.

To produce $1^\triangle$ base UP, the lens must be decentred $c_V = 0.25$ cm

$$= 2.5 \text{ mm}$$

and since the lens is negative, the decentration must be DOWNWARDS, i.e., $c_V = 2.5$ mm down.

To produce $1^\triangle$ base IN, the lens must also be decentred 2.5 mm, but this time OUTWARDS, i.e., $c_H = 2.5$ mm OUT.

The optical centre of the lens must therefore occupy a position 2.5 mm below and 2.5 mm to the temporal side of the standard optical centre position.

This lens, after laying off, should have the appearance shown in *Figure 43.1b.*

In the following experiment, a number of spherical lenses are to be marked ready for glazing to the instructions accompanying the lenses.

Apparatus

Box of uncut spherical lenses together with instructions giving their powers and the specified decentration or prismatic effect; neutralizing set; centring machine or crossline chart; protractor; lens marking equipment.

127

Procedure

(1) Using the centring machine (or crossline chart), mark the optical centre of each lens.

(2) Sort out the lenses by neutralization to match the instruction sheets.

Where decentration is specified

(3) Place the lens on the protractor with its front surface uppermost and its optical centre over the centre of the protractor (intersection of 90 and 180 meridians of the protractor).

(4) Using the guide scales on the protractor, move the lens so that its optical centre lies at the specified distance from the centre of the protractor. For example, if the decentration which is required is 3 mm inwards for the right eye, move the lens to the right until the optical centre lies 3 mm to the right of the intersection of the 90 and 180 meridians at the centre of the protractor.

(5) Hold the lens firmly in this position upon the protractor and draw the horizontal cutting line along the 180 meridian of the lens, following the 180 meridian of the protractor.

(6) Without disturbing the position of the lens on the protractor, draw a shorter vertical cutting line along the vertical meridian of the lens, following the 90 meridian of the protractor.

(7) Indicate which eye the lens is intended for by marking R or L in the upper temporal quadrant of the lens and by drawing an arrowhead near the nasal end of the horizontal cutting line (as shown in *Figure 43.1*).

Where prismatic effect is specified

If the prismatic effect which is to be produced is stated and not the decentration itself, this latter quantity must first be determined from $c = \dfrac{P}{F}$ as shown in example (2).

When the amount and direction of the decentration has been established, the experiment may proceed from step (3).

Note. – Remember the rule, 'decentre a positive lens in the same direction as the prism base required, but a negative lens in the opposite direction to the prism base required.'

(8)   Before the lens is sent to the glazing department, it is necessary to ensure that the uncut lens size is large enough to include the finished lens size when the cutting lines lie in their usual positions for the lens shape. If we assume that the lenses are to be glazed round in shape and that the standard optical centre position is to coincide with the datum centre, then the largest diameter round eye which can be obtained from each of the marked uncuts can be determined from the distance from the intersection of the cutting lines to the closest point on the lens periphery. The maximum finished lens size is clearly twice this distance.

The student should determine this maximum finished lens size for each of his marked uncuts.

Experiment 44
RECORDING THE COMPLETE PRESCRIPTION OF EDGED DECENTRED LENSES

Theory

The complete prescription of an edged lens involves recording not only the lens power and axis direction but also the prismatic effect at the standard optical centre position of the lens. In this experiment we assume that the standard optical centre position coincides with the datum centre of the lens.

The prescription of each lens should first be recorded and the positions of the optical centre and datum centre marked. The position of the optical centre in relation to the datum centre (i.e., the decentration of the optical centre) can then be measured and the prismatic effect introduced at the datum centre calculated.

The following examples should make this last procedure clear.

Examples

(1)   Rx. L. + 4.00 DS. Optical centre lies 5 mm to nasal side of datum centre.

The prismatic effect at the datum centre is found from the decentration relationship $P = cF$.

We have $P = 0.5 \times 4$
$$= 2^\triangle.$$

The lens has been decentred inwards so that the base direction of this prism is also IN. The complete prescription is therefore L. + 4.00 DS $\circeq 2^\triangle$ base IN.

130

(2) Rx. R. − 2.00/ − 4.00 × 90. Optical centre lies 5 mm above and 5 mm to nasal side of datum centre.

The principal powers of the lens are − 2.00 D along the vertical meridian and − 6.00 D along the horizontal.

Vertical prismatic effect $P_V = c_V F_V$
$$= 0.5 \times 2$$
$$= 1^\triangle \text{ base DOWN}$$

(since negative lens has been decentred inwards).

Horizontal prismatic effect $P_H = c_H F_H$
$$= 0.5 \times 6$$
$$= 3^\triangle \text{ base OUT}$$

(since negative lens has been decentred upwards).

The complete prescription is R. − 2.00/ − 4.00 × 90 ∘ $1^\triangle$ base DOWN and $3^\triangle$ base OUT.

(3) Rx. R. + 3.00/ + 2.00 × 60. Optical centre lies 5 mm to temporal side of datum centre.

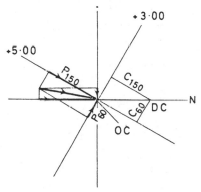

Figure 44.1. Graphical construction to obtain prismatic effect of lens for right eye + 3.00/ + 2.00 × 60 decentred out 5 mm along 180

The principal powers of the lens are + 3.00 D along 60 and + 5.00 D along 150. We must resolve the decentration along these meridians. The simplest method is by scale drawing (*Figure 44.1*).

It can be seen from *Figure 44.1* that the 5 mm outward decentration is equivalent to 2.5 mm DOWN and OUT along 60 and 4.33 mm UP and OUT along 150.

131

TABLE 44.1

Lens No.	Eye	Prescription	Decentration and direction	Prismatic effect
Example 1	L	+4.00	5 mm IN	2$^\triangle$ base IN
Example 2	R	−2.00/−4.00 × 90	5 mm UP and 5 mm IN	1$^\triangle$ base DOWN and 3$^\triangle$ base OUT
Example 3	R	+3.00/+2.00 × 60	5 mm OUT	2.3$^\triangle$ base UP at 169 or 0.44$^\triangle$ base UP and 2.24$^\triangle$ base OUT

The prismatic effect along 60, P_{60},
$$= c_{60} F_{60}$$
$$= 0.25 \times 3$$
$$= 0.75^{\triangle} \text{ base DOWN at } 60.$$

The prismatic effect along 150, P_{150},
$$= c_{150} F_{150}$$
$$= 0.433 \times 5$$
$$= 2.17^{\triangle} \text{ base UP at } 150.$$

These two prismatic effects may now be compounded into a single resultant effect and, finally, the single resultant effect may be resolved into vertical and horizontal components. The methods used are precisely the same as those given in Experiment 42, but since we have already constructed the 60 and 150 meridians of the lens in *Figure 44.1*, the new graphical work may be performed on the same diagram. Thus, drawing the prisms to scale and completing the rectangle, we find the resultant prismatic effect to be $2.3^{\triangle}$ base UP at 169, and resolving this effect along the vertical and horizontal meridians, $0.44^{\triangle}$ base UP and $2.24^{\triangle}$ base OUT.

The complete prescription is therefore R. $+ 3.00/ + 2.00 \times 60$, $0.44^{\triangle}$ base UP and $2.24^{\triangle}$ base OUT.

Apparatus

Box of edged decentred lenses; neutralizing set; centring machine or crossline chart; protractor; ruler.

Procedure

(1) Find the power and axis direction (if astigmatic) of each lens and mark optical centre. Whether the lens is for the right or the left eye should be self-evident.

(2) Mark the datum centre of each lens and measure the vertical and horizontal distances from this to the optical centre. Note the direction of these decentrations.

(3) Calculate the prismatic effect at the datum centre of each lens.

Record your results as shown in Table 44.1.

Experiment 45
NEUTRALIZATION OF BROKEN LENSES

Theory

The replacement of broken lenses is part of the service offered by an optician, and the determination of the lens power, form, axis direction and position of the optical centre is his responsibility. If the lens (or a remnant of the lens) is still held in the frame, the procedure is exactly the same as for a glazed frame. Usually, however, the broken lens is brought in in pieces and the following procedure should then be adopted.

Apparatus

Set of broken lenses in envelopes; neutralizing set; crossline chart; lens measure; transparent adhesive tape.

Procedure

Neutralize one lens at a time. Replace each piece in envelope before beginning with the next. Handle broken pieces with care!

(1)   Select largest piece of broken lens and determine whether spherical or astigmatic. If astigmatic, mark one of the principal meridians by the rotation test.

(2)   Neutralize the broken piece.

(3)   Using the lens measure, determine the form of the lens.

(4)   Arrange all the broken pieces together so that the original lens shape can be determined. If the lens is astigmatic, select the piece which lies diametrically opposite to the piece which you have already

neutralized. Mark the same principal meridian of this piece as marked on the largest piece (i.e., 'plus axis' or 'minus axis').

(5) Using strips of transparent adhesive tape, stick the pieces together so that the complete lens may be picked up in one piece. Use the minimum amount of tape.

(6) Mark the optical centre of the lens.

(7) Place the lens on the protractor, front surface uppermost, and record the cylinder axis direction in standard notation and the position of the optical centre in relation to the datum centre.

(8) Measure datum lens size and note the type of edge (e.g., bevelled or grooved). Identify the lens shape.

Record your results as shown below.

Lens No.	Sph.	Cyl.	Axis	Form	Dec.	Lens size and shape	Edge

Experiment 46
TO RECORD THE MINIMUM SPECIFICATION OF A PAIR OF SPECTACLES

Theory

It is sometimes necessary to duplicate a given pair of spectacles. The purpose of this experiment is to record the essential details of the lenses and the frames so that an identical pair of spectacles can be supplied by a prescription house. A suitable duplicate frame may be considered to be one in which only minor adjustments by the optician are necessary to copy exactly the measurements of the original frame. The lens specification should include, in addition to the powers and orientation, the lens form and thickness.

Apparatus

Focimeter, lens measure, thickness calipers, frame rule, prescription order forms, pairs of spectacles.

Procedure

(1)   Adjust the focimeter for your own use. Record the powers of the lenses and measure any vertical prismatic effect. Record the reading addition (if any).

(2)   Adjust each lens so that the focimeter target is central in the graticule, at least horizontally, and using the marking device dot the optical centre. (If the focimeter does not include a marking device, it will be necessary to do this with a centring machine.)

(3)   Measure the centration distance and if necessary calculate any horizontal prismatic effect.

(4)   Using the lens measure, record the form of the lens. It is only necessary to state the base curve if the lens is spherical or the sphere curve if it is toroidal. If the lens is a fused bifocal, record the base curve; if a solid bifocal, record the DP curve.

(5)   Using thickness calipers, record the centre thickness (i.e., the thickness at the optical centre of the lens). If the lens is prismatic and the optical centre does not lie on the lens area, record the thin edge substance. In this last case, state where the thickness has been measured.

(6)   Record any segment dimensions.

(7)   State the type and tint (if any) of the lens and, if special, its edge form.

(8)   State the type, colours and material of the spectacle frame. If the frame appears to be a hand-made special, state the thickness of the material and type of joints.

(9)   Measure the datum lens size and datum centre distance. The bridge measurements which should be specified depend upon the type of bridge as follows.

Regular bridge	*Pad bridge*
Height	Distance between lenses
Projection	Position and size of pads
Apical radius	Distance between pad centres
Base and depths	

(10)   Record the frontal width and the joint angle. State the type and total length of the sides. Measure length to bend (or length to tangent if curl sides).

Any of the above details which do not have a particular space allocated on the prescription form should be written in the space for special instructions.

Experiment 47
VERIFICATION OF COMPLETED PRESCRIPTIONS

Theory

The complete prescription, on return from the workshop, must be checked against the original specification. In addition to the correct powers, cylinder axis direction, centration and form, the quality of the materials and workmanship must be checked. Errors or defects should be noted carefully and concisely so that if the work is returned to the prescription house for correction, there can be no doubt as to the validity and cause of complaint.

The relevant British Standards should be consulted for a guide to the permitted tolerances.

Apparatus

Verification sets with prescription orders, lens measure, focimeter, strain tester, frame rule, thickness calipers.

Procedure

(1) Check the lenses first. Check type and tint if specified, then as follows.

Lens powers.
Cylinder axis direction.
Reading addition.
Prism power and base setting.
Position of the optical centre and segment location.
Lens form (lens measure).
Lens thickness (thickness calipers).

(2) When you are satisfied with the optical details of the lens, check the following.

Lens surfaces for defects.
Lens material for defects.
Strain.
Lens shape and size.
Quality of edge, etc.

(3) *Frame details*. Check the type and colour of the frame and its material. Verify the frame measurements. Pay particular attention to the following details.

Plastics frames

Lens tight in rims. No gaps. Grooves central.
Rims not burnt, warped or twisted.
Rims of even thickness.
Sides and front in alignment.
Sides open easily. Screws not loose.

Metal frames

Joints closed. Lenses tight without strain.
No gaps or packing.
Screw-heads not damaged.
Side screws tight.
Swivel pads moving.
Metal free from plier marks.
Sides and front in alignment.

Rimless frames

Quality of edge. No facets, starring, etc.
Screws tight but no strain. Heads undamaged.
Straps snugly against edge and surface of lens.
Sleeves on spring bar fittings.
Top bar properly spaced from lens and conforming to lens shape.
Sides and front in alignment.

Supra frames

Cord not frayed or cracked.
Cord holes in same positions.
Knot well into countersink. No sharp cord ends should be felt.
Quality of edge. No starring or chips.
Grooves follow lens edge centrally.
Lenses do not rock in mount.
No threads trapped under cord.
Sides and front in alignment.

Experiment 48
OPTICAL BENCH MODEL OF A VERTEX
POWER MEASURING INSTRUMENT

Theory

We require to measure the vertex powers of ophthalmic lenses. Due to the finite thickness of ophthalmic lenses, the vertex power differs from the equivalent power. If the lens is very thin, the vertex power is virtually the same as the equivalent power.

Figure 48.1 shows the equivalent focal length f' of a lens of finite thickness d. The back vertex power F'_V is defined as $\dfrac{1}{f'_V}$ and the equivalent focal power F is defined as $\dfrac{1}{f'}$, f'_V and f' being measured in metres. If the lens is very thin so that d is zero, $f' = f'_V$.

Figure 48.2 shows the formation of the image of an object placed within the focal length of a convex lens and the equation $xx' = -f'^2$ is derived.

Note that the distances x and x' are measured from the first and second focal points respectively. Thus in *Figure 48.2*, x is positive and x' is negative. Hence the negative signs in equations (1) and (2), since h' and h are positive.

The principle of the focimeter is based on Newton's equation $xx' = -f'^2$, and a model of the instrument is to be constructed with the aid of an optical bench and accessories. This model instrument is to be calibrated and used to measure the vertex powers of ophthalmic lenses.

Apparatus

Optical bench; light source; pinhole aperture standard lens of known focal power (say + 7 D); circular aperture to act as a positioning stop; telescope; lens of unknown back vertex power.

Procedure

Adjust the telescope so that it is focused for infinity. Place the standard lens at a fixed position on the optical bench. Place the source behind the pinhole aperture and locate the pinhole aperture at the first

Figure 48.1. f' is the equivalent focal length of the lens, thickness d. If f' is expressed in metres, then $1/f' = F$, the equivalent focal power. f'_V is the back vertex focal length. If f'_V is expressed in metres, then $1/f'_V = F'_V$, the back vertex power. If the lens is infinitely thin so that d is virtually zero, then $F = F'_V$

focal point F_0 of the standard lens. When the aperture is at F_0, light emerging from the standard lens will be parallel and will be focused by the telescope and seen clearly by an emmetropic observer with accommodation relaxed. Repeat this observation several times and obtain the mean, and record the position of F_0.

Place the telescope on the other side of the lens, repeat the above procedure and locate the position of the second focal point F'_0. Now arrange the accessories on the optical bench in the following order (*Figure 48.3*): source, pinhole aperture at F_0, standard lens at its fixed position, positioning stop at F'_0, and telescope. Check that these are correctly positioned by looking through the telescope; the point source

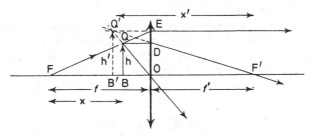

Figure 48.2. Object BQ, size h, is imaged as a virtual image B'Q', size h'. F and F' are the first and second focal points of the lens. The distances from the first focal point to the object and from the second focal point to the image are called extra-focal distances and given the symbols x and x' respectively. From the diagram:

$$Magnification\ m = \frac{h'}{h} = \frac{Q'B'}{QB}\ ,\ but\ QB = DO$$

$$= \frac{Q'B'}{DO}$$

$$= \frac{F'B'}{OF'},\ since\ triangles\ Q'B'F'\ and\ DOF'\ are\ similar$$

$$= -\frac{x'}{f'} \qquad \qquad \ldots (1)$$

(Note that m is positive since image is erect; in diagram, f' is positive but x' is negative, hence negative sign is necessary because of sign convention.)

$$Also\ magnification\ m = \frac{h'}{h} = \frac{Q'B'}{QB} = \frac{EO}{QB}\ since\ EO = Q'B'$$

$$= \frac{OF}{FB} \qquad \begin{array}{l} since\ triangles\ EOF\ and\ QBF \\ are\ similar \end{array}$$

$$= \frac{-f}{x} \qquad \qquad \ldots (2)$$

From equations (1) and (2):

$$\frac{-x'}{f'} = \frac{-f}{x}$$

$$or - xx' = -ff',\ but\ -f = f',$$

$$\therefore\ -xx' = f'^2$$

$$or\ xx' = -f'^2$$

143

due to the pinhole aperture should be imaged at infinity and will therefore be seen clearly.

If a lens of unknown focal power is placed against the positioning stop at F'_0, the image of the source at F_0 when viewed through the telescope will be blurred. If, as in *Figure 48.3*, the lens is convex, the pinhole aperture must be moved from F_0 a distance x to some new position B so that its image is again seen clearly in the telescope. If the

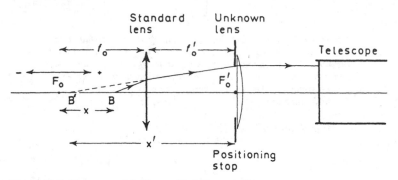

Figure 48.3. Compare with Figure 48.2. F_0 and F'_0 are the first and second focal points of the standard lens. Target B, distance x from F_0, is imaged by standard lens at B', distance x' from F'_0. The lens of unknown power is placed in the second focal plane of the standard lens passing through F'_0. If the object B is imaged at infinity after refraction by the standard lens and the unknown lens, the point B' coincides with the focal point of the unknown lens and x' is numerically equal to the back vertex focal length f'_V of the unknown lens

lens had been of negative focal power, the source and pinhole aperture would have had to be moved in the opposite direction. Note that the front surface of the unknown lens must be furthest away from the standard lens, otherwise the front vertex power will be measured.

From *Figure 48.3*,

$$F'_0 B' = x' = -f'_V, \text{ hence } xx' = -xf'_V = -f'^2_0$$

Since $f'_V = \dfrac{1}{F'_V}$, $\quad F'_V = \dfrac{x}{f'^2_0}$ (x and f'_0 must be in metres)

$$= \dfrac{x}{f'^2_0} \times 1,000 \text{ (x and } f'_0 \text{ in millimetres)}.$$

Hence F'_V = x times a constant, since f'_0 is constant, so the back vertex power F'_V is directly proportional to the movement x of the pin-

144

hole aperture. If $F'_V = 1$ D, then $1 = \dfrac{1,000x}{f'_0{}^2}$, therefore the amount of movement of the target is $\dfrac{f'_0{}^2}{1,000}$ mm per dioptre.

Exercises

(1) Calibrate the instrument experimentally in millimetres per dioptre by using three trial case lenses. Compare with the calculated value. Record the results.

Use the instrument to determine and record the back vertex power of the unknown spherical lenses. More accurate results will be obtained if (a) a yellow filter is used in front of the source and (b) a concentric circle of pinhole apertures surrounds the central pinhole aperture.

(2) Measure the back vertex power of six unknown spherical lenses.

(3) Measure the back vertex power of six unknown astigmatic lenses. Note that each pinhole aperture is imaged as a short focal line which is perpendicular to the direction of the meridian producing it.

Experiment 49
THE FOCIMETER

Theory

The focimeter is an optical instrument for measuring the vertex power of a combination of trial case lenses or the vertex power of a spectacle lens. It is designed to measure prisms, prismatic effects and the axis direction of astigmatic lenses and usually has a marking device.

All instruments are liable to error. In this experiment a series of lenses of accurately known power and axis direction are measured with the focimeter and a curve of the readings is plotted. This is compared with the actual known power of the lenses and a calibration curve is obtained. This calibration curve can then be used to correct errors (if any) of the instrument.

Apparatus

Focimeter to be calibrated; neutralizing set with lenses whose back vertex power is very accurately known; manufacturer's instructions in the use of the focimeter; graph paper.

Procedure

(1) Read the manufacturer's instructions.
(2) Correct adjustment of eyepiece (the observer should wear his distance prescription).
    (a) Set the dioptre scale at any position other than zero.
    (b) Withdraw the eyepiece to its greatest extent.
    (c) Move eyepiece slowly inward and observe the graticule.

(d) Cease movement of eyepiece when graticule is seen distinctly.

(e) Adjust the dioptre scale until the target is seen distinctly. The scale should now read zero.

Keep both eyes open during step (2). These operations ensure that the target is viewed with accommodation relaxed.

(3) Plot a dioptre scale (same units) on the y and x axis of the graph paper as shown.

On the horizontal scale, plot the reading given by the focimeter. On the vertical scale, plot the known power of the lens. If there are no

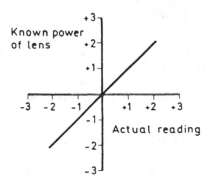

Figure 49.1

errors in the instrument, the calibration curve will be a straight line making an angle of 45° with either axis. Draw this line.

From the neutralizing set, take out the + 0.25 D sph. and determine its power by use of the focimeter. If possible, your partner should give you other lenses from the neutralizing set without your observing the engraved power of the rim; this ensures independent observations. When this has been done, the roles can be reversed. Thus each person determines his own results. Plot the results and hence the calibration curve.

Axis check

The test cylinder should have its flat edge exactly parallel to the cylinder axis. Place this on the lens platform. If the direction of the focal lines is determined to be 90° or 180°, the 0°−180° line of the axis scale will be parallel to the lens platform. Reverse the test lens and check.

Determine very accurately the axis direction of the lenses in the finished spectacles, which should be at an oblique axis by a method other than the focimeter. Compare with the focimeter reading.

Prism scale

This is usually in the form of a tangent scale. Determine the power of the prisms in the neutralizing set with the focimeter. Draw a calibration curve.

Sensitivity of the instrument

(1)   Power scale. Measure say a + 8.00 D sphere. Note whether a variation of 0.12 D on the power scale (+ 8.00 D ± 0.12 D) can be observed. Determine the minimum change on the power scale which causes the target to become just indistinct. Record this value and compare it with any observations made later on other makes of focimeter.

(2)   Axis direction. Measure say a + 1.00 D cylinder axis 180. Rotate the axis scale ± 10° and note how the target becomes indistinct. Determine the minimum change in axis direction which causes the target to become just indistinct. Record this value and compare it with observations made later on other makes of focimeter.

(3)   Obtain two plano-prisms whose power in prism dioptres is accurately known and which differ by $0.25^\triangle$, say $3.0^\triangle$ and $3.25^\triangle$. Measure these on the focimeter and record the results. Estimate whether you could read the scale to (a) $0.12^\triangle$ and (b) $0.06^\triangle$. Obtain a + 1.00 D sph. which has been decentred 5 mm. Measure with the focimeter the prism due to decentration and compare this result with the calculated result, using $P = cF$.

Experiment 50
EFFECTIVE POWER OF A THIN LENS

Theory

Figure 50.1 shows parallel light incident on a thin positive lens, focal power F dioptres, which is brought to a focus distant f' metres from the thin lens.

At d metres from the lens, the vergence of the light is by definition

$$\frac{1}{f'-d} = \frac{1/f'}{1-d/f'} = \frac{F}{1-dF}$$

This vergence is termed the effective power of the lens at a distance d metres from the lens.

Let F_d represent the effective power in dioptres.

Then $F_d = \dfrac{F}{1-dF}$

This experiment gives two methods of investigating this last equation.

METHOD 1

Apparatus

Thin positive lens of unknown power F (approx. 4 D or 5 D); distant target; ruler; neutralizing set.

Procedure

Place the neutralizing lens not in contact with the unknown lens but at a distance d metres from it. Apply the transverse test. If there is a with movement, decrease, and if there is an against movement, increase the power of the neutralizing lens, keeping d constant. When applying the transverse test, both lenses must be moved an equal transverse distance. When there is no movement, the power opposite in sign to that of the

Figure 50.1. Parallel light is converged by the lens, and immediately after refraction by the lens has a vergence of F dioptres where F is the focal power of the lens. At a distance d metres from the lens the vergence of the light is no longer F dioptres; hence a lens placed d metres from the lens F dioptres will require to have a focal power F_d dioptres for the light to emerge parallel. F_d is numerically the effective power of the lens, focal power F, at distance d metres

Figure 50.2

neutralizing lens will be F_d, the effective power of the unknown lens at a distance d metres from the lens. If the unknown lens has a power of approximately 4 D or 5 D, an initial value of d could be approximately 2 cm. Increase the neutralizing power in steps of 0.50 D and obtain corresponding values of d. Plot $1 + dF_d$ as abscissa against F_d as ordinate. The slope of the graph will give the focal power in dioptres of the unknown lens power F.

This experiment requires precise measurement of d and accurate neutralization. It will help if you have a partner to assist in measuring d. Note that the distant target will appear slightly magnified. This is due to the combination of lenses in *Figure 50.2* acting as a Galilean telescope.

METHOD 2

Apparatus

Optical bench and accessories; collimator; telescope; neutralizing set.

Procedure

Arrange the accessories in the following order from left to right on the optical bench: source, collimator, lens of unknown focal power, then neutralizing lens distant d metres away, followed by the telescope.

Adjust the telescope so that it is focused for a distant object. Look through the telescope and move the neutralizing lens towards the lens of unknown focal power F until the image from the collimator is just blurred, then withdraw the lens until it is just clear. Measure d and note the power of the neutralizing lens. Increase the neutralizing lens in steps of 0.50 D and obtain corresponding values of d. Plot a graph as before. If a collimator is not available, use a distant object.

To prove that the slope of the graph gives the focal power F,

$$F_d = \frac{F}{1 - dF}$$

$$F_d (1 - dF) = F$$

$$F_d = F + dF.F_d$$

$$= F (1 + dF_d)$$

$$\frac{F_d}{1 + dF_d} = F$$

Hence a graph of F_d against $1 + dF_d$ will have a slope of value F.

Record your result as follows.

1	*2*	*3*	*4*
Power of neutralizing lens	F_d	*d metres*	$1 + dF_d$

Columns 1 and 2 have the same magnitude but are opposite in sign.

Experiment 51
VERTEX POWERS OF SPECTACLE LENSES

Theory

When the form and thickness of a spectacle lens are taken into account, it is not sufficient to add together the surface powers of the lens in order to discover its refracting properties. The quantity $F = F_1 + F_2$, the sum of the surface powers, is often referred to as the 'thin lens power' of the lens. The total effect of a lens, however, depends also on its thickness and its refractive index.

Figure 51.1 illustrates a positive lens whose thickness is such that it cannot be neglected when considering the focal properties of the lens. The horizontal line which intersects the lens surfaces F_1 and F_2 at the points A_1 and A_2 represents the optical axis of the lens. The centres of curvature of the lens surfaces lie on this line. The point A_1 is called the front vertex of the lens. The point A_2 is the back vertex. The distance $A_1 A_2 = t$ is the axial thickness of the lens. If light of wavelength 587.56 nm (helium d) is incident, parallel to the optical axis, on the front surface of the lens and close to the optical axis, it is refracted by the lens to focus at the point F'. This point is called the back vertex focus of the lens, and the distance $A_2 F' = f'_V$ (f'_V in metres) is the *back vertex power* of the lens, F'_V. Similarly, F is the front vertex focal point of the lens for light incident upon the back surface. $A_1 F$ is the front vertex focal length, f_V, and the reciprocal of f_V is the *front vertex power* F_V.

Only when the lens is symmetrical (i.e., $F_1 = F_2$) are the front and back vertex powers the same. In spectacle optics we are usually concerned only with the back vertex power of the lens. However, when we measure the power of a curved lens by neutralization, the neutralizing lens is held in contact with the front surface of the lens under test.

Here we are measuring the front vertex power, and for this reason this power is often referred to as the *neutralizing power* of the lens.

Figure 51.1. The lens has surface powers F_1 and F_2, physical thickness t, and vertices A_1 and A_2. Parallel light from the left is focused at F', distance f'_V from vertex A_2. Parallel light from the right is focused at F, distance f_V from vertex A_1. If f'_V and f_V are measured in metres, the reciprocals of these distances give the magnitude of the back vertex power F'_V and the front vertex power F_V

The back vertex power of a lens may be found from the equation

$$F'_V = \frac{F_1 + F_2 - t/n\, F_1 F_2}{1 - t/n\, F_1}$$

F_1 and F_2 are the front and back surface powers, t is the axial thickness, and n the refractive index of the lens.

The front vertex power is given by

$$F_V = \frac{F_1 + F_2 - t/n\, F_1 F_2}{1 - t/n\, F_2}$$

Note the similarity of these equations. The numerator is the same in each. When the surface powers, thickness and refractive index of a lens are known, its vertex powers may be calculated from the above equations.

Examples

(1) A positive lens has surface powers $F_1 = +10.00$ D, $F_2 = +5.00$ D. Its axial thickness t = 6 mm and it is made from glass of refractive index 1.5. Calculate the vertex powers of the lens.

153

Front vertex power:

$$F_V = \frac{F_1 + F_2 - t/n\,F_1F_2}{1 - t/n\,F_2} \quad \text{(t must be in metres)}$$

$$= \frac{10 + 5 - 0.004 \times 10 \times 5}{1 - 0.004 \times 5}$$

$$= \frac{14.80}{0.98}$$

$$= +15.10 \text{ D.}$$

Back vertex power:

$$F'_V = \frac{F_1 + F_2 - t/n\,F_1F_2}{1 - t/n\,F_1}$$

$$= \frac{10 + 5 - 0.004 \times 10 \times 5}{1 - 0.004 \times 10}$$

$$= \frac{14.80}{0.96}$$

$$= +15.42 \text{ D.}$$

(2)   A lens whose surface powers are $F_1 = +15.00$ D and $F_2 = -5.00$ D has an axial thickness of 7.5 mm and is made in glass $n = 1.5$. Calculate its vertex powers.

Front vertex power:

$$F_V = \frac{F_1 + F_2 - t/n\,F_1F_2}{1 - t/n\,F_2}$$

$$= \frac{15 - 5 + 0.005 \times 15 \times 5}{1 + 0.005 \times 5}$$

$$= \frac{10.375}{1.025}$$

$$= +10.12 \text{ D.}$$

Back vertex power:

$$F'_V = \frac{F_1 + F_2 - t/n\,F_1F_2}{1 - t/n\,F_1}$$

$$= \frac{15 - 5 + 0.005 \times 15 \times 5}{1 - 0.005 \times 15}$$

$$= \frac{10.375}{0.925}$$

$$= + 11.21 \text{ D.}$$

(3) An astigmatic lens has surface powers

$$\frac{+ 10.00 \text{ DC} \times 90 / + 14.00 \text{ DC} \times 180}{- 4.00 \text{ DS}}$$

It is made in glass n = 1.5 and has an axial thickness of 6 mm. Calculate its back vertex power.

Base curve meridian

$$F'_V = \frac{F_1 + F_2 - t/n \, F_1 F_2}{1 - t/n \, F_1}$$

$$= \frac{10 - 4 + 0.004 \times 10 \times 4}{1 - 0.004 \times 10}$$

$$= \frac{6.16}{0.96}$$

$$= + 6.42 \text{ DC} \times 90$$

Cross curve meridian

$$F'_V = \frac{F_1 + F_2 - t/n \, F_1 F_2}{1 - t/n \, F_1}$$

$$= \frac{14 - 4 + 0.004 \times 14 \times 4}{1 - 0.004 \times 14}$$

$$= \frac{10.224}{0.944}$$

$$= + 10.83 \text{ DC} \times 180$$

$$F'_V = + 6.42 \text{ DC} \times 90 / + 10.83 \text{ DC} \times 180$$

$$= + 6.42 \text{ DS} / + 4.41 \text{ DC} \times 180.$$

In the following experiment the surface powers F_1 and F_2 are to be recorded by means of a lens measure, the thickness measured, and the front and back vertex powers calculated from the formulae given above.

Apparatus

Box of high powered positive lenses; lens measure; thickness calipers. (Logarithm tables or slide rule are also required.)

Procedure

(1) By means of the lens measure, record the front and back surface power of the lens. (Check lens measure for zero error.)

(2)　Mark the position of the optical centre and measure the thickness at this point. (Check calipers for zero error.)

(3)　Calculate the front and back vertex powers from the equations given above.

The results are most easily verified by means of the focimeter.

Experiment 52
FRONT AND BACK VERTEX POWERS;
SURFACE POWERS OF A THICK LENS
IN AIR

Theory

Figure 52.1 shows parallel light incident on the front surface of a thick plano-convex lens in air. After being refracted by the two surfaces of the lens, it is brought to a focus at the point F'. Parallel light is incident on the back surface of the lens, and after refraction by the two surfaces of the lens it is brought to a focus at F. A_1 and A_2 are the vertices of the lens surfaces. The purpose of this experiment is to compare the vertex powers and the 'thin lens power' which is simply $(F_1 + F_2)$.

Apparatus

Positive meniscus lens, plano-convex lens and equiconvex lens, all of high power; lens measure; neutralizing set; focimeter.

Procedure

(1)   Measure the surface powers F_1 and F_2 of each lens
(2)   Measure the front and back vertex powers by neutralization. When the neutralizing lens is in contact with the front surface of the lens, the front vertex power is obtained. When the neutralizing lens is in contact with the back surface of the lens, the back vertex power is obtained. It will therefore not be possible to obtain accurately by neutralization the back vertex power of the meniscus lens.
(3)   Measure the vertex powers of each lens by the focimeter. Record your results as follows.

Lens type	Surface powers		Vertex powers by neutralization		Vertex powers by focimeter		Thin lens power
	F_1	F_2	F_V	F'_V	F_V	F'_V	$F_1 + F_2$
Meniscus							
Plano convex							
Equiconvex							

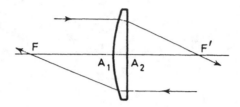

Figure 52.1. Front and back vertex focal length of a thick lens in air.

$A_1 F$ = front vertex focal length.
$A_2 F'$ = back vertex focal length.

Front vertex power of lens $F_V = -1/f_V$ (f_V in metres).
Back vertex power of lens $F'_V = 1/f'_V$ (f'_V in metres)

Note that the thin lens power is the power of each lens if it were very thin.

(4) Compare in each case F_V and F'_V.

(5) Compare in each case F'_V and $F_1 + F_2$.

(6) Prove that the difference between the back vertex power of the lens (F'_V) and the thin lens power ($F_1 + F_2$) is given by

$$F'_V - (F_1 + F_2) = \frac{tF_1^2}{n - tF_1}$$

Repeat the experiment using a negative meniscus lens of high power and a plano-concave lens of high power.

Experiment 53
MARKING AND SETTING BY MEANS
OF THE FOCIMETER

Theory

Most focimeters incorporate a marking device which enables the optical centre and axis direction of the lens under test to be marked. This device takes the form of three spring-loaded pointers which, when not in use, rest on an ink-soaked pad which lies in a well attached to the body of the instrument. When the marking device is brought into operation, the pointers lift from the pad and swivel into line with the optical system of the instrument; the three pointers then lie in a horizontal line parallel to the lens platform. Further operation of the control presses the pointers against the lens, which is clamped in its usual position on the lens rest. The marking device thus places three dots on the lens, the straight line joining the dots lying parallel to the line of the lens rest.

Two different procedures may be adopted to mark an astigmatic lens. The device may be used only to mark the optical centre and cylinder axis direction, followed by hand setting of the lens in the usual manner by means of a protractor. If this method is adopted, the power of the lens is checked in the usual way and then the lens is rotated so that its axis lies parallel to the 180 meridian of the focimeter's protractor. The lens is then adjusted horizontally until the focimeter target lies at the centre of the graticule and the marking device is operated. The two outer dots on the lens then represent the cylinder axis direction and the centre dot coincides with the optical centre of the lens.

Alternatively, the marking device may be used to indicate the horizontal cutting line and the standard optical centre position. This method eliminates the need for hand setting and may be used when the

159

lens is to be edged by an automatic machine. Here the lens power is checked in the normal way and then the lens is rotated until its cylinder axis lies along the prescribed meridian. When the cylinder axis has been correctly set, the lens may be finally adjusted vertically and horizontally until the target lies at the centre of the graticule and the marking device is brought into operation. The two outer dots now represent the horizontal cutting line and the centre dot represents the optical centre of the lens.

When marking spherical lenses, it is only necessary to adjust the lens so that the target lies at the centre of the graticule. When the marking device is operated, the centre dot here represents the optical centre.

The focimeter marking device is very useful for marking and setting a lens which incorporates a prismatic element. The lens may be adjusted in the clamp until the target lies across the prescribed prism power. The centre dot then represents the standard optical centre position, and if the lens includes a cylindrical element and the second method described above is adopted, there is no need to mark the lens any further.

The marking device must not be operated unless there is a lens in position in the clamp.

Apparatus

Focimeter which incorporates a marking device; box of uncut lenses which have to be set to given prescriptions; protractor.

Procedure

(1) Adjust the focimeter for your own use. Place a lens in position on the rest and hold it with the clamp.

(2) Check the power of the lens.

(3) Holding the lens against the stop, release the clamp sufficiently to enable you to move the lens.

(4) If the lens is spherical, adjust its position until the target lies at the centre of the graticule.

If the lens is astigmatic, rotate it until the given cylinder axis lies along the 180 meridian and adjust it horizontally until the target lies at the centre of the graticule.

(5) Operate the marking device.

(6) Remove the lens and place it on the protractor. Lay off in the usual way, using the outer dots to indicate the cylinder axis direction (if the lens is astigmatic).

(7)   Replace the lens in the focimeter with your cutting line parallel to the lens rest. Re-operate the marking device. The three new dots should all lie on your cutting line provided that you have correctly re-centred the lens.

Experiment 54
THE NEUTRALIZATION AND
SPECIFICATION OF BIFOCALS

Theory

The complete identification of a bifocal lens involves the recognition of the type, form, powers, centration and segment location of the lens. Recognition of the bifocal type requires familiarity with the available bifocal designs, which may be broadly grouped into four categories as follows.

(1) Split bifocals.
(2) Cement bifocals.
(3) Fused bifocals.
(4) Solid bifocals.

The form of the bifocal (and an estimate of its power) may be obtained by means of a lens measure. It is necessary only to give the base curve of the lens, or in the case of solid bifocals the DP curve. If the bifocal is solid or cemented in type, the lens measure may also be used to obtain a good estimate of the reading addition, since this is the difference between the DP and RP curves of the lens.

The distance portion power and axis direction may be found by neutralization or by means of the focimeter. In this experiment we will assume the use of neutralizing lenses. The reading addition (or Add) may also be found by neutralization (or by the focimeter) since this is the difference between the reading portion power and the distance power. The Add is the difference between the vertex powers of the surface on which the segment is located. Thus if the segment is incorporated upon the back surface of the lens, the Add is the difference between the back vertex powers of the DP and RP, but if the segment is incorporated upon the front surface of the lens, the Add is the difference between the front vertex powers.

The centration of the distance portion is found by locating the distance optical centre just as for single vision lenses. The centration of the reading portion is a little more difficult and will not be considered in this experiment. (*See* Experiment 55.)

The size and position of the segment can be recorded from the following information.

Segment diameter (round segments) (Figure 54.1)

The diameter of the circle of which the segment forms a part.

Segment height (Figure 54.1)

The vertical distance from the segment top to a horizontal line tangential to the lens periphery at its lowest point.

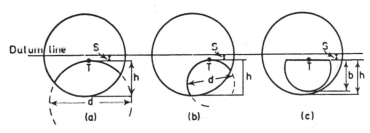

Figure 54.1. Segment location terminology. T = segment top; s = segment top position; d = segment diameter; h = segment height; b = segment depth

Segment top position (Figure 54.1)

The vertical distance of the segment top above or below the datum line of the lens.

Geometrical inset (Figure 54.2)

The horizontal distance between vertical lines which pass through the distance centration point (i.e., the distance optical centre or the point where it would be placed in the absence of prescribed prism) and the mid-point of the segment.

163

Note. – In the case of crescent segments, it is usual to give the geometrical inset as the horizontal distance FE measured 15 mm below the distance centration point (*Figure 54.2b*).

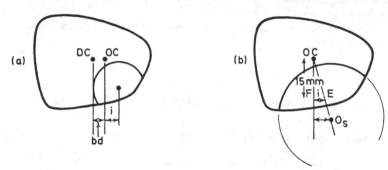

Figure 54.2. Segment location terminology. i = geometrical inset; bd = bodily decentration; OC = distance centration point (and in the absence of any prescribed prismatic effect, the position of the distance optical centre); DC = datum centre

Figure 54.3

Segment drop or cutting instruction (Figure 54.3)

The vertical distance from the segment top to the distance centration point.

In addition the following information might be required.

Segment depth (Figure 54.1c)

The vertical distance from the segment top to a horizontal line tangential to the segment at its lowest point, the segment nowhere extending to the lens periphery.

164

Segment size

A specification consisting of the segment diameter and the segment depth, usually given only with shaped segments.

Bifocal segment positions are specified by stating the segment diameter (or size in the case of shaped segments), the segment height or segment top position, the geometrical inset and the segment drop (or 'cut' as it is sometimes called). For example, the specification

$$22 \times 18 \times 2\frac{1}{2}, \text{ drop } 5$$

indicates that the segment diameter is 22 mm, the segment height 18 mm, the geometrical inset 2.5 mm and the segment drop 5 mm. If the finished lens size is 40 mm round, the segment top position is 2 mm below datum and the specification might be written

$$22 \times 2 \text{ bel} \times 2\frac{1}{2}, \text{ drop } 5.$$

It should be noted that the second dimension gives the vertical position of the segment and the third dimension represents the inset.

Apparatus

Edged bifocal lenses; neutralizing set; centring machine or crossline chart; lens measure; ruler.

Procedure

(1)   Mark the optical centre and the cylinder axis (if astigmatic) of the bifocal lens.

(2)   Neutralize the distance portion of the lens. It may help to obscure the segment area with the thumb during this process.

(3)   Neutralize the reading portion. The Add is almost always simply a spherical component, so that subtraction of the distance power from the reading power immediately gives the Add. If the distance portion is astigmatic, the following procedure may be followed. Neutralize the DP along the cylinder axis meridian. Record this power as the sphere of the distance portion. Neutralize the RP along the same meridian and record this power as the DP sphere plus the Add. The Add is then this last power minus the DP sphere. (But note third paragraph under 'Theory' above.)

(4)   Record the form of the lens by means of the lens measure. State the base curve or, in the case of a solid or cement bifocal, the DP curve.

TABLE 54.1

Lens No.	Distance prescription	Add	Type	Form	Bodily dec.	Segment				
						Diameter or size	Height	Inset	Drop	Top position
1	+ 5.00 / − 0.50 × 5	2.00	Fused	− 6.00 base	2 in	20	16	2	4	2½ below

(5) Measure the segment diameter (or segment size for shaped segments), the segment height and the geometrical inset (refer to *Figures 54.1* and *54.2*). Assume that the distance centration point coincides with the datum centre of the lens.

(6) Measure the segment drop *(see Figure 54.3)* and also any horizontal decentration of the distance optical centre.

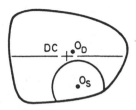

Figure 54.4

Note. — The geometrical inset is the horizontal distance from the distance optical centre to the mid-point of the segment (or a point 15 mm below the distance optical centre in the case of a crescent segment). Any decentration of the distance optical centre in the horizontal meridian from the datum centre is referred to as bodily decentration.

(7) Measure the vertical box dimension of the lens and subtract the segment height from half this dimension to obtain the segment top position.

The bifocal lens shown in *Figure 54.4* has the following specification:

$$22 \times 16 \times 2$$

distance optical centre decentred 2 in bod. Segment top position = 2½ below. Segment drop = 4 mm below.

Record your results as shown in Table 54.1

Experiment 55
PRISMATIC EFFECT AT THE NEAR
VISUAL POINT OF A BIFOCAL LENS

Theory

A bifocal lens may be considered to be made up from two separate components: a main lens which incorporates the distance prescription, and a segment lens whose power is equal to the reading addition *(Figure 55.1a)*.

When the power of each of these components is known together with the position of their optical centres, the prismatic effect at any point in the segment can be calculated. It is convenient to consider the prismatic effect of each component lens separately.

Suppose that a bifocal lens has the power + 2.00 DS Add 2.00 D for near. The segment is 22 mm in diameter and is of the invisible variety, i.e., its optical centre — considered as a separate lens — coincides with its geometrical centre. The segment top lies 5 mm below the distance optical centre and the segment has been inset 2.5 mm. It is required to calculate the total prismatic effects at a point within the segment area 10 mm below the distance optical centre and 2.5 mm inwards.

We have power of main lens = + 2.00 D; power of segment lens = + 2.00 D.

Vertical meridian

The near visual point lies 10 mm below the distance optical centre, so that c = 1 cm *(see Figure 55.1)*. The segment top lies 5 mm below the distance centre, and so the near visual point must lie 5 mm below the segment top. The radius of the segment is 11 mm, so y = 6 mm or 0.6 cm.

Horizontal meridian

The segment lens has been inset by the same amount as the near visual point, so it introduces no horizontal prismatic effect. The

Figure 55.1. O_D is the optical centre of the main or distance lens. O_S is the optical centre of the segment lens. The near visual point NVP is c cm below the distance optical centre and y cm above the segment optical centre. c_H is the horizontal separation of the optical centres of the main lens and segment lens

horizontal prismatic effect at the near visual point is thus that due to the main lens alone. $c_H = 0.25$ cm.

The prismatic effects are found from the relationship $P = cF$.

	Vertical	*Horizontal*
Prism due to main lens	$2.00^\triangle$ base UP	$0.50^\triangle$ base OUT
Prism due to segment	$1.20^\triangle$ base DOWN	
Total prismatic effect at near visual point	$0.80^\triangle$ base UP	$0.50^\triangle$ base OUT

Examples

The following examples should also be worked through. The near visual point is assumed to be 10 mm below and 2.5 mm inwards from the distance optical centre. In some cases the segment is not inset by the same amount as the near visual point.

169

(1) R. − 4.00 DS Add 1.50 38 segment, inset 2.5 mm, segment top 4 mm below distance optical centre.

	Vertical	Horizontal
Prism due to main lens	4.00 △ base DOWN	1.00 △ base IN
Prism due to segment	1.95 △ base DOWN	–
Total prismatic effect at NVP	5.95 △ base DOWN	1.00 △ base IN

(2) L. + 2.00 DS Add 2.50 30 segment, inset 4.5 mm, segment top 3 mm below distance optical centre.

	Vertical	Horizontal
Prism due to main lens	2.00 △ base UP	0.50 △ base OUT
Prism due to segment	2.00 △ base DOWN	0.50 △ base IN
Total prismatic effect at NVP	0	0

(3) L. + 3.00/ + 2.00 × 180 Add 1.00 45 segment, inset 2.5 mm, segment top 5 mm below distance optical centre.

	Vertical	Horizontal
Prism due to main lens	5.00 △ base UP	0.75 △ base OUT
Prism due to segment	1.75 △ base DOWN	–
Total prismatic effect at NVP	3.25 △ base UP	0.75 △ base OUT

(4) R. + 2.00/ + 2.00 × 60 Add 2.00 38 segment, inset 1.5 mm, segment top 2 mm below distance optical centre.

	Vertical	Horizontal
Prism due to main lens (see Experiment 42)	2.72 △ base UP	1.74 △ base OUT
Prism due to segment	2.20 △ base DOWN	0.20 △ base OUT
Total prismatic effect at NVP	0.52 △ base UP	1.94 △ base OUT

In the following experiment, the prismatic effects at the near visual point of various bifocal lenses are to be found by calculation and the results checked by neutralization at the near visual point, using prisms.

PRISMATIC EFFECT AT NEAR VISUAL POINT OF A BIFOCAL LENS

Apparatus

Edged invisible bifocal lenses; neutralizing set (including a range of prisms, preferably in $\frac{1}{2}^\triangle$ steps); centring machine or crossline chart; ruler.

Procedure

(1) Neutralize the distance portion of the lens and find the reading addition.

(2) Carefully mark the optical centre of the lens.

(3) Draw a horizontal line, parallel to the datum line of the lens, through the distance optical centre *(see Figure 55.1b)*.

(4) Mark the optical centre of the segment lens considered as a separate entity. For round invisible segments, this will be the geometrical centre of the segment. Draw a vertical line through this point.

(5) Draw a horizontal line tangential to the segment top, and mark a point in the segment area 6 mm below this horizontal line and on the vertical line which passes (or would pass in the case of crescent segments) through the segment centre.

(6) The lens should now be similar in appearance to the one illustrated in *Figure 55.1b*.

Measure the distances c, c$_H$ and y shown in *Figure 55.1b*.

(7) Use these distances to calculate the prismatic effect at the near visual point as shown in the preceding examples.

(8) Holding the lens before the crossline chart, place neutralizing prisms over the segment area, the powers of which are the same as the prismatic effects calculated in step (7), but their bases placed in the opposite direction (e.g., if the prismatic effects found in step (7) are $1^\triangle$ UP and $2^\triangle$ OUT, the neutralizing prisms should be $1^\triangle$ DOWN and $2^\triangle$ IN). The crosslines should be unbroken when the near visual point lies on the line joining the centre of the crosslines and the eye.

Note. – For simplicity, this experiment should be restricted to low power bifocal lenses for ease of observation.

171

Experiment 56
MARKING AND SETTING BIFOCALS

Theory

The marking and setting, or laying off, procedure for uncut bifocal lenses follows the method used in earlier experiments for single vision lenses except that in addition to the correct orientation of the cylinder axis (if the lens is astigmatic) and optical centre of the main lens, the bifocal segment must also be positioned. As with single vision lenses, the glazing department requires to know only which is the front surface of the lens and its correct orientation.

Apparatus

Uncut bifocal lenses together with their prescriptions and segment location; neutralizing set; centring machine or crossline chart; protractor; ruler; lens marking equipment.

Procedure

(1) Sort out the lenses by neutralization to match the prescription sheets.

(2) Mark the optical centre and cylinder axis direction of the main lens.

(3) Outline the segment periphery by placing a series of dots along the dividing line on the segment surface of the lens. This will facilitate the location of the segment on the protractor.

(4) Indicate the geometrical centre of the segment with a small

172

dot. In the case of crescent segments, indicate a point on the vertical line passing through the distance centration point and the geometrical centre of the segment 15 mm below the distance centration point *(see Figure 54.2b)*.

(5)   Place the lens, front surface uppermost, on the protractor and adjust so that the cylinder axis lies along the prescribed meridian and the centre of the segment lies to the nasal side of the 90 meridian of the protractor by the amount of the inset required. If the lens is spherical, the inset may be obtained by rotating the lens about its optical centre until the centre of the segment occupies the correct position*. In the case of crescent segments, the inset is obtained when the point 15 mm below the distance centration point lies to the nasal side of the 90 meridian by the prescribed amount†.

(6)   Draw a vertical cutting line on the lens, following the 90 meridian of the protractor. This establishes the correct inset and cylinder axis orientation.

(7)   Move the lens along the 90 meridian of the protractor, keeping the vertical cutting line parallel to this meridian until the segment top lies at the prescribed distance below (or above) the 180 meridian of the protractor. Draw the horizontal cutting line on the lens, following the 180 meridian of the protractor.

(8)   Indicate which eye the lens is intended for by drawing an arrowhead near the nasal end of the horizontal cutting line and by marking R or L in the upper temporal quadrant of the lens.

Note. – When a pair of bifocal lenses is being marked, the segment location of each lens should be checked by holding the lenses together, their convex surfaces in light contact, with the cutting lines over each other. The segments should then also appear to be exactly over each other (assuming, of course, that the segment location of each is the same).

---

*Except with straight-top segments, when the horizontal top must remain parallel with the datum line of the lens.

†The distance optical centre should now be correctly positioned.

Experiment 57
FUSED BIFOCALS

Theory

The fused bifocal consists in principle of a flint lens fused into a crown lens as shown in *Figure 57.1*. The refractive index of the flint lens is about 1.654 in practice; we will denote this by n_s. The refractive index of the crown lens is 1.523; we will denote this by n. The reading addition is made up partly by the difference between the contact surface powers and partly by the difference between the front surface powers over the different glasses.

From *Figure 57.2* the contact surface power required to produce a given reading addition can be deduced. The power of the contact surface *in situ* will be denoted by F_{con}. Usually we are more concerned with the power of the depression curve F_c in air. The reading addition is denoted by A.

It can be seen from *Figure 57.2* that the total reading addition is made up from the addition due to the front surface $(F_3 - F_1)$ and the power of the contact surface (F_{con}),

i.e., $A = F_3 - F_1 + F_{con}$.

Now $F_3 = (n_s - 1) R_1$, $F_1 = (n - 1) R_1$, and $F_{con} = (n - n_s) R_c$,

$\therefore A = (n_s - n) R_1 + (n - n_s) R_c$

$= \dfrac{(n_s - n)}{(n - 1)} F_1 - R_c (n_s - n)$

or $R_c = \dfrac{F_1}{(n - 1)} - \dfrac{A}{(n_s - n)}$

174

FUSED BIFOCALS

The power of the contact surface in air, F_c, $= (n - 1) R_c$,

$$\therefore F_c = F_1 - \frac{A(n-1)}{(n_s - n)} = F_1 - A.k$$

where k is the fused bifocal blank ratio $\dfrac{n-1}{n_s - n}$

Substituting 1.523 for n and 1.654 for n_s, we find

$$k = \frac{0.523}{0.131} = 4 \text{ very nearly, so that } F_c = F_1 - 4A.$$

We now see that $A = \dfrac{F_1}{4} - \dfrac{F_c}{4}$, and so the Add due to the front

surface is $\dfrac{F_1}{4}$ (assuming k = 4) and the Add due to the contact surface

is $\dfrac{F_c}{4}$

Figure 57.1

Figure 57.2

Figure 57.1. Cross-sectional view of a fused bifocal lens. A flint button of high refractive index is fused into a countersink on the crown blank

Figure 57.2. The front surface of the fused bifocal lens has the same curvature over the main lens and the segment. The refractive index of the main lens is denoted by n, and the refractive index of the segment (shaded in diagram) by n_s Since n_s is greater than n, the focal power of the front segment surface is F_3 and that of the main lens is F_1, and F_3 is greater than F_1. Hence the contribution to the reading addition of the front surface is $F_3 - F_1$. F_{con} is the focal power of the contact surface separating the segment from the main lens. The total reading addition A is given by the amount provided by the front surface plus the amount provided by the contact surface. Hence $A = (F_3 - F_1) + F_{con}$.
If the contact surface were plano, A would be given by $(F_3 - F_1)$.
F_C is the focal power of the contact surface in air

175

Suppose a fused bifocal has a depression curve of −4.00 D. The Add due to the contact surface is + 1.00 D. If it is required to make up a total addition of + 2.00 D, the front surface power must also be + 4.00 D. In short,

$$A = \frac{F_1}{4} - \frac{F_c}{4}$$

$$= \frac{4}{4} + \frac{4}{4}$$

$$= + 2.00 \text{ D.}$$

Alternatively, if a finished fused bifocal lens has a front surface power of + 10.00 D and reading addition of + 1.00 D, the Add due to the front surface is $\frac{10.00}{4}$ or + 2.50 D and the contact surface must be contributing − 1.50 D. Since the Add due to the contact surface is $F_{con} = - \frac{F_c}{4}$, the depression curve in air $F_c = - 4F_{con} = + 6.00$ D.

Examples

(1) The prescription + 1.50 /+ 1.00 × 90 Add 2.50 is made up as a fused bifocal on a − 5.50 D base curve using glasses n = 1.523, n_s = 1.654. Find the power of the depression curve.

The form of the lens is $\dfrac{+ 8.00 \text{ DS}}{- 5.50 \text{ DC} \times 90/ - 6.50 \text{ DC} \times 180}$

$$k = \frac{0.523}{0.131} = 4$$

$$F_c = F_1 - Ak$$

$$= 8 - 2.50 \times 4$$

$$= - 2.00 \text{ D.}$$

The power of the depression curve is − 2.00 D.

(2) The prescription − 6.00 DS/ + 2.00 DC × 30 Add 2.00 is to be made up in fused bifocal form using glasses n = 1.5 and n_s = 1.6. If the base curve is − 8.00 DC, find the power of the depression curve.

176

The form of the lens is $\dfrac{+4.00 \text{ DS}}{-8.00 \text{ DC} \times 30/-10.00 \text{ DC} \times 120}$

$$k = \frac{0.5}{0.1} = 5$$

$$F_c = F_1 - Ak$$
$$= 4 - 2 \times 5$$
$$= -6.00 \text{ D.}$$

The power of the depression curve is -6.00 D.

Assuming that the component flint and crown lenses which make up the reading portion of a fused bifocal are thin, the powers of these two elements can be determined from *Figure 57.3.*

Figure 57.3. F_2 is the focal power of the second surface of the main lens. F_S is the focal power of the segment element in air. F_B is the focal power of the lens portion bounded by the contact surface and the second surface of the main lens and $F_B = F_C + F_2$

The power of the back element F_B is equal to $F_c + F_2$.

Since $F_c = F_1 - Ak$,
we have $F_B = F_1 - Ak + F_2$
$$= F - Ak$$

where F is the distance portion power ($F_1 + F_2$).

The power of the segment element F_S can be determined as follows. The total power in the reading portion $= A + F = F_S + F_B$,

i.e., $F_S = A + F - F_B$,
or since $F_B = F - Ak$,
$$F_S = A (k + 1).$$

It can be seen that the powers of these two elements are quite independent of the form of the lens. Thus the fused bifocal -3.00 DS Add 2.00, made up in glasses which produce a blank ratio of 4, would have the following component elements.

Segment element $F_S = A(k + 1) = 2 \times 5 = + 10.00$ D.
Back element $\quad F_B = F - Ak = -3 - 8 = -11.00$ D.

Adding together these two elements, we obtain the power of the reading portion, -1.00 DS.

The following experiments are designed to verify the above relationships. They require the use of the component elements of a fused bifocal. These should be separate as shown in *Figure 57.3*. The k ratio for the component glasses should be given.

Apparatus

Fused bifocal components (back and segment elements with a common contact surface); focimeter; lens measure.

Procedure

(1) Neutralize the distance portion of the back element (F).

(2) With the segment element in position, neutralize the reading portion $(A + F)$.

(3) Subtract the distance power from the reading portion power to obtain the Add (A).

(4) Calculate the power of the back and segment elements from

$$\left. \begin{array}{l} F_B = F - Ak \\ \text{and } F_S = A(k + 1) \end{array} \right\} \text{ k should be given.}$$

(5) Verify the powers of these elements by neutralization.

(6) Using the lens measure, record the front surface power distance portion, F_1.

(7) Calculate the power of the depression curve on the back element from $F_c = F_1 - Ak$.

(8) Verify the power by the lens measure.

(9) Divide the powers found in steps (6) and (7) by the k ratio to obtain $\dfrac{F_1}{k} - \dfrac{F_c}{k}$.

(10) Evaluate $\dfrac{F_1}{k} - \dfrac{F_c}{k}$ (take care with the sign of F_c).

What does this give? Prove this from first principles.

(11) Evaluate $\dfrac{F_1 - F_c}{A}$

What does this give?

Record your results as shown in the table below.

Lens No.	Distance portion (F)	Add (A)	F_B (F − Ak)	F_S A (k + 1)	F_1	F_c $(F_1 − Ak)$	$\dfrac{F_1}{k}$	$\dfrac{F_c}{k}$	$\dfrac{F_1}{k}$	$\dfrac{F_c}{k}$	$\dfrac{F_1 − F_c}{A}$

Compatible flint series

It is possible to obtain a complete range of reading additions by employing a single depression curve and varying the refractive index of the segment glass. This system demands the availability of a full series of compatible flint glasses of suitable physical properties but has the advantage that it is no longer necessary to maintain a large number of tools in order to work the depression curves.

Some fused bifocal manufacturers have switched their production method entirely to a compatible flint system. Others use just three or four different glasses and a reduced number of depression curves.

In order to find the refractive index of the flint glass which is required to produce a given addition, we write the expression, $F_c = F_1 − Ak$, in the form

$$k = (F_1 − F_c) / A,$$

and since k is given by $(n − 1) / (n_s − n)$, we find

$$n_s = n + \frac{(n − 1)}{(F_1 − F_c)} A.$$

For a given crown glass major, n is constant, so that the difference between the crown and flint glass refractive indices is given by the term

$$\frac{(n − 1)}{(F_1 − F_c)} A.$$

If we now arrange for $F_1 − F_c$ to be constant throughout the range we would have a fully compatible flint series.

For example, suppose that additions from +0.75 D to +3.00 D are required and we use the following combinations of front curves and depression curves

DP curve F_1	depression curve F_c
+8.00	−2.00
+6.00	−4.00
+4.00	−6.00

179

the quantity $(n-1) / (F_1 - F_c)$ becomes 0.0523 (assuming that $n = 1.523$), and the compatible flint range is given by

$$n_s = 1.523 + 0.0523A.$$

The required series of flint glasses would be

Add	n_s	Add	n_s
+0.75	1.562	+2.00	1.628
+1.00	1.575	+2.25	1.641
+1.25	1.588	+2.50	1.654
+1.50	1.601	+2.75	1.667
+1.75	1.614	+3.00	1.680

Experiment 58
SURFACE POWER AND RADIUS OF SURFACING LAPS

Theory

The focal power in dioptres of a surface separating glass, refractive index n, and air is given by

$$F = \frac{(n-1)}{r}$$

where F is the focal power in dioptres and r is the radius of curvature of the surface in metres.

Exercises

(1) If F = 4 D, n = 1.523 (spectacle glass), calculate r.

$$F = \frac{(n-1)}{r}$$

$$4 = \frac{0.523}{r}$$

$$\frac{0.523}{4} = r \text{ metres}$$

$$\frac{523}{4} = r \text{ mm}$$

$$130.75 = r \text{ mm}$$

Now draw an arc of radius 131 mm. Select the template used to check a spectacle tool to give a surface power of 4 D. Place the template against the arc. Do they match?

(2) Repeat for F = + 6 D. (*Answer:* r = 87.16 mm. Draw arc radius 87 mm.)

(3) Repeat for + 5 D, but glass is now flint n = 1.65.

$$\text{Hence } + 5 = \frac{(1.65 - 1)}{r}$$

(*Answer:* r = 13 cm.)

Draw an arc with the calculated radius and select the template to check a spectacle tool to give a surface power of 5 D. Do they match? If not, why not?

(4) An 8 D spectacle tool is used to work the surface of a flint lens n = 1.65. What is the surface power of the flint lens. (*Answer:* almost 10.)

Note. — If compasses are not available, draw around the templates and measure the actual radius of the template. Use a fine pointed pencil with care.

Experiment 59
SAG CALCULATIONS

Theory

In Experiment 19 it was shown that the relationship between the sag of a curve, s, for a given lens diameter, 2y, the radius of curvature of the surface under consideration being denoted by r, is

$$s^2 + y^2 = 2rs.$$

Writing this relationship in the form $s^2 - 2rs + y^2 = 0$ and solving the quadratic, we obtain (disregarding the plus sign before the radical):

$$s = r - \sqrt{(r^2 - y^2)} \qquad \ldots (1)$$

Equation (1) could be derived immediately from the geometry of *Figure 19.1* where s = AC, y = CD and r = OA = OD, for in the right-angled triangle OCD, $OC = \sqrt{(OD^2 - CD^2)} = \sqrt{(r^2 - y^2)}$. Since AC = OA − OC, we can write immediately,

$$s = r - \sqrt{(r^2 - y^2)}$$

Since $r = \dfrac{n-1}{F}$ where F is the optical power of the surface, we can write

$$s = \frac{n-1}{F} - \sqrt{\left[\left(\frac{n-1}{F}\right)^2 - y^2\right]} \qquad \ldots (2)$$

Substituting 1.523 for n and the lens diameter d (= 2y), if d is given in millimetres we can write

$$s = \frac{523}{F} - \sqrt{\left[\left(\frac{523}{F}\right)^2 - \frac{d^2}{4}\right]} \qquad \ldots (3)$$

Equation (3) gives the sag of a curve F at the lens diameter d in millimetres. It is an exact relationship, and sag tables are compiled from this equation.

It was also shown in Experiment 19 that when s is small compared with y and r, we can write approximately:

$$s = \frac{y^2}{2r}$$

Again substituting $\dfrac{n-1}{F}$ for r, we find

$$s = \frac{y^2 F}{2(n-1)}$$

or expressing s and y in millimetres,

$$s = \frac{y^2 F}{2,000(n-1)} \qquad \ldots (4)$$

This is an approximate equation for s. It provides adequate solutions only when it is used for low power surfaces at small diameters.

Exercises

(1) Calculate the radius of curvature of a surface of power 10.00 D separating glass, n = 1.523, from air.

Draw an arc with the calculated radius and construct two chords 50 mm and 60 mm in length. Measure the sags s for these two chords.

(2) Repeat for a surface of 20.00 D and chords 40 mm and 30 mm in length.

(3) Calculate these sags by means of equations (4) and (3). Check the calculations against the accompanying worked solutions.

Solutions

Approximate

$$s = \frac{y^2 F}{2,000(n-1)}$$

$$y = 25 \text{ mm}$$

$$F = 10 \text{ D}$$

183

$$n = 1.523$$

$$s = \frac{25^2 \times 10}{2,000 \times 0.523}$$

$$= \frac{6,250}{1,046}$$

$$= 5.98 \text{ mm.}$$

Accurate

$$s = \frac{523}{F} - \sqrt{\left[\left(\frac{523}{F}\right)^2 - \frac{d^2}{4}\right]}$$

$$= \frac{523}{10} - \sqrt{\left[\left(\frac{523}{10}\right)^2 - \frac{50^2}{4}\right]}$$

$$= 52.3 - \sqrt{(52.3^2 - 625)}$$

$$= 52.3 - \sqrt{(2,735 - 625)} \text{ to four-figure accuracy}$$

$$= 52.3 - \sqrt{2,110}$$

$$= 52.3 - 45.93$$

$$= 6.37 \text{ mm.}$$

Approximate

$$y = 30 \text{ mm}$$

$$F = 10 \text{ D}$$

$$n = 1.523$$

$$s = \frac{30^2 \times 10}{2,000 \times 0.523}$$

$$= \frac{9,000}{1,046}$$

$$= 8.6 \text{ mm.}$$

Accurate

$$s = \frac{523}{10} - \sqrt{\left[\left(\frac{523}{10}\right)^2 - \frac{60^2}{4}\right]}$$

$$= 52.3 - \sqrt{(2{,}735 - 900)}$$
$$\doteq 52.3 - \sqrt{1{,}835}$$
$$= 52.3 - 42.84$$
$$= 9.46 \text{ mm.}$$

Approximate

$$s = \frac{y^2 F}{2{,}000\,(n - 1)}$$

$$y = 20 \text{ mm}$$
$$F = 20 \text{ D}$$
$$n = 1.523$$

$$s = \frac{20^2 \times 20}{2{,}000 \times 0.523}$$

$$= \frac{8{,}000}{2{,}000 \times 0.523}$$

$$= \frac{4}{0.523}$$

$$= 7.65.$$

Accurate

$$s = \frac{523}{F} - \sqrt{\left[\left(\frac{523}{F}\right)^2 - \frac{d^2}{4}\right]}$$

$$= \frac{523}{20} - \sqrt{\left[\left(\frac{523}{20}\right)^2 - \frac{1{,}600}{4}\right]}$$

$$= 26.15 - \sqrt{(683.8 - 400)}$$
$$= 26.15 - 16.84$$
$$= 9.31 \text{ mm.}$$

185

Approximate

$$s = \frac{y^2 F}{2,000 \, (n - 1)}$$

$y = 15 \text{ mm}$

$F = 20 \text{ D}$

$n = 1.523$

$$= \frac{225 \times 20}{2,000 \times 0.523}$$

$$= \frac{2.25}{0.523}$$

$$= 4.3 \text{ mm.}$$

Accurate

$$s = \frac{523}{F} - \sqrt{\left[\left(\frac{523}{F} \right)^2 - \frac{d^2}{4} \right]}$$

$$s = \frac{523}{20} - \sqrt{\left[\left(\frac{523}{20} \right)^2 - \frac{900}{4} \right]}$$

$$= 26.15 - \sqrt{(683.8 - 225)}$$

$$= 26.15 - 21.42$$

$$= 4.73 \text{ mm.}$$

Experiment 60
THE JALIE PRISM PROTRACTOR

Theory

The Jalie prism protractor was primarily designed to find the prismatic effect at any point on a cylindrical lens. With the instrument, the prismatic effect exerted by a plano-cylinder can be found quite rapidly without the use of a graphical construction. The principle of the instrument is as follows.

It was shown in Experiment 42 that the vertical and horizontal prismatic effects at any point on a plano-cylinder are given by $P_V = AQ\ F_{cyl}$ and $P_H - QR\ F_{cyl}$ *(Figure 60.1)*. It should be apparent from *Figure 60.1* that $AQ = AR \cos \theta$ and $QR = AR \sin \theta$.

In a circle of radius AR *(Figure 60.2)*, the radius subtending the angle θ, we find $AR \cos \theta = c$ and $AR \sin \theta = s$. The vertical and horizontal prismatic effects at the point R are thus $P_V = c\ F_{cyl}$ and $P_H = s\ F_{cyl}$ respectively, c and s being expressed in centimetres. The instrument allows the distance AR to be found from one setting of the cursor and then the distances c and s from a second setting.

The protractor can also be used for compounding and resolving prism powers and for finding the decentration necessary to produce a prescribed prismatic effect.

The instrument consists of two separate components, the 'protractor' which bears the main scale and a 'cursor' capable of being placed in any position relative to the main scale.

PRISMATIC EFFECT OF A CYLINDER

Procedure

(1) Place the horizontal axis of the cursor on the protractor along the axis meridian of the given cylindrical component. The face of the

187

protractor at this stage represents the lens, and the perpendicular distance of any point on the lens from the cylinder axis can be read from the scale on the cursor.

Figure 60.1. *Vertical prismatic effect at point* $R = AQ.F_{cyl}$. *Horizontal prismatic effect at point* $R = QR.F_{cyl}$

Figure 60.2. *Circle of radius AR.* $c = AR \cos \theta$; $s = AR \sin \theta$

(2)   Find on the upper half of the main scale of the protractor the point at which the cylinder axis in question meets a circle whose radius is equal to the perpendicular distance found in step (1). The vertical distance from this point to the 180 degrees meridian of the main scale is the *horizontal* decentration, which when multiplied by the power of the cylinder gives the *horizontal* prismatic effect. The horizontal distance of this point from the 90 degrees meridian of the main scale is the *vertical* decentration required, which when multiplied by the power of the cylinder gives the *vertical* prismatic effect.

The base directions of these prismatic effects are easily found as follows.

188

For plus cylinders the cylinder axis represents the base of the prismatic effect. Its position – during step (1) – in relation to the point at which the prismatic effect is being calculated immediately shows the base direction of the prismatic effect.

With minus cylinders, the cylinder axis represents the position of the apex of the prismatic effect in relation to the point. Obviously for minus cylinders the base is in the opposite direction.

Figure 60.3a–d demonstrates the base direction of the prismatic effect at the point R in each of the diagrams.

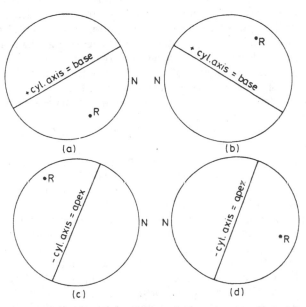

Figure 60.3. (a) Right eye plus cylinder prismatic effect at R = base UP & OUT resolving to base UP and base OUT. (b) Left eye plus cylinder prismatic effect at R = base DOWN & IN resolving to base DOWN and base IN. (c) Right eye minus cylinder prismatic effect at R = base UP & OUT resolving to base UP and base OUT. (d) Left eye minus cylinder prismatic effect at R = base DOWN & OUT resolving to base DOWN and base OUT

Examples

(1) Find the prismatic effect at a point 6 mm below and 4 mm inwards from the optical centre of the lens L. + 2.00 DS/ + 2.00 DC × 120.

189

Prism due to sphere (by inspection)

$$= 1.2^\triangle \text{ UP}$$
$$= 0.8^\triangle \text{ OUT.}$$

Prism due to cylinder

Place the horizontal axis of the cursor along 120 degrees on the protractor and read by the scale on the cursor the perpendicular distance of the point (6 mm below and 4 mm inwards from the zero of the main scale) from the cylinder axis (= 6.4 mm). Notice also that the cylinder axis lies *upward* and *outward* in relation to the point. Now on the main scale find the point where the 120 degrees meridian meets a circle of radius 6.4 mm (by interpolation between the 6 mm and 7 mm circles). (The bare vertical axis of the cursor will be found to help here since it can be slid over to pass through this point.)

The horizontal distance of this point from the 90 degrees meridian = 3.2 mm = 0.32 cm.

The vertical distance of this point from the 180 degrees meridian = 5.6 mm = 0.56 cm.

The vertical prismatic effect due to the cylinder = horizontal distance X power of cylinder = 0.32 X 2 = $0.64^\triangle$.

The horizontal prismatic effect due to the cylinder = vertical distance X power of cylinder = 0.56 X 2 = $1.12^\triangle$.

Since it is a positive cylinder and its axis lies upward and outward from the point at which the prismatic effect is being found — the axis representing the position of the prism base in relation to the point — the base direction of the prismatic effect is base UP and OUT.

Hence the prismatic effect exerted by the cylinder = $0.64^\triangle$ base UP and $1.12^\triangle$ base OUT. Adding the prism due to the sphere, the total prismatic effect at a point 6 mm below and 4 mm inwards from the optical centre of the lens L. + 2.00 DS/ + 2.00 DC X 120 = $1.84^\triangle$ base UP and $1.92^\triangle$ base OUT.

(2)   Find the prismatic effects at a near visual point 11 mm below and 2.5 mm inwards from the optical centre of the lens R. + 6.00/ − 4.00 X 140.

Prism due to sphere (by inspection)

$$= 6.6^\triangle \text{ base UP}$$
$$= 1.5^\triangle \text{ base OUT.}$$

Prism due to cylinder

Place the horizontal axis of the cursor along 140 degrees on the main scale. Notice that the cylinder is negative and its axis lies *upward* and *inward* in relation to the near visual point. Hence the cylinder is producing prism base DOWN and OUT at the point.

Read off the perpendicular distance of the near visual point from the cylinder axis = 6.9 mm.

On the main scale, find the point where the 140 degrees meridian meets a circle of radius 6.9 mm. The horizontal distance of this point from the 90 degrees meridian = 5.2 mm = 0.52 cm.

The vertical distance of this point from the 180 degrees meridian = 4.4 mm = 0.44 cm.

The vertical prismatic effect due to the cylinder = horizontal distance X power of cylinder = $0.52 \times 4 = 2.08^\triangle$ base DOWN.

The horizontal prismatic effect due to the cylinder = vertical distance X power of cylinder = $0.44 \times 4 = 1.76^\triangle$ base OUT.

Adding the prism due to the sphere, the total prismatic effect at the near visual point = $4.52^\triangle$ base UP and $3.26^\triangle$ base OUT.

COMPOUNDING AND RESOLVING PRISMS

Procedure

The following diagrams and examples will make the procedure for compounding and resolving prisms with the aid of the protractor quite clear.

Examples

(1) Compound $6^\triangle$ base UP and $8^\triangle$ base IN into a single prismatic effect for the right eye (*Figure 60.4*).

(2) Compound $2\frac{1}{2}^\triangle$ base DOWN and $3\frac{1}{2}^\triangle$ base IN into a single prismatic effect for the left eye (*Figure 60.5*).

(3) Resolve $4^\triangle$ base UP and IN at 30 into vertical and horizontal components (*Figure 60.6*).

Note. – Shorthand multiplication can always be used to evaluate prismatic effects due to cylinders, since any cylinder power containing quarter dioptres can be expressed as a fraction with a denominator of 4, e.g., 1.75 cyl. = 7/4 cyl., etc.

Figure 60.4. Example 3. Compounding prisms by
means of the protractor. $6^\triangle$ base UP ≏ $8^\triangle$ base IN
≡ $10^\triangle$ base UP at 37

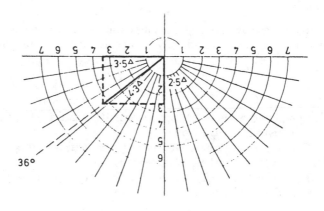

Figure 60.5. Example 4. Compounding prisms by means of
the protractor. $2\frac{1}{2}^\triangle$ base DOWN ≏ $3\frac{1}{2}^\triangle$ base IN ≡ 4.3 base
DOWN at 36

192

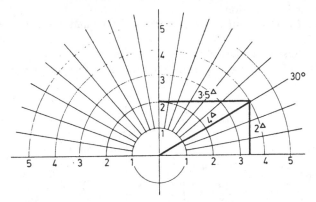

Figure 60.6. Example 5. Resolving prisms by means of the protractor. $4^\triangle$ base UP at 30 $\equiv 2^\triangle$ base UP $\circ$ 8.5 base IN

DECENTRATION TO PRODUCE PRISMATIC EFFECTS

Procedure

The prism protractor can also be used to find the decentration necessary to produce a given prismatic effect, although in these days of focimeters with marking devices the occasions when this procedure is required are likely to be few. However, the instrument eliminates the need for an accurate graphical construction, since the prisms and decentrations involved can be compounded and resolved on the main scale of the protractor, following the principles of the graphical construction.

The method will be illustrated by an example, the rules for the graphical construction being given first.

Example

Find the decentration required to produce $4^\triangle$ base UP and $2^\triangle$ base OUT with the lens for the right eye + 4.50 /+ 2.50 × 70.

Graphical solution

The graphical solution is illustrated in *Figure 60.7.*
The rules for construction are as follows.

193

(1) Construct origin and principal meridians of lens showing powers and orientation.

(2) Draw in prisms to scale (OW and OV) and construct resultant point Z.

(3) Resolve prisms along the principal meridians of the lens (ZY and ZX) by dropping perpendiculars from Z to the principal meridians.

Figure 60.7

(4) Measure ZX and ZY and calculate the decentrations necessary to produce them:

$$\text{Use } c = \frac{P}{F}$$

The resultant decentrations OQ and OP are shown in *Figure 60.7*.

(5) Compound decentrations OQ and OP into a single decentration OR (not shown in *Figure 60.7*) and resolve OR into vertical and horizontal components RV and RH.

RV = vertical decentration required.
RH = horizontal decentration required.

In the present example,

$ZX = 3.1^\triangle$ UP and IN at 70.

$ZY = 3.3^\triangle$ UP and OUT at 160.

$OQ = \dfrac{3.1}{4.5}$ cm = 6.9 mm UP and IN at 70.

$OP = \dfrac{3.3}{7}$ cm = 4.7 mm UP and OUT at 160.

The directions for the decentrations are found from the rule: 'To obtain prism by decentration, decentre a positive lens in the same direction as the prism base required and decentre a negative lens in the opposite direction.' Compounding OQ and OP, the final result obtained is RV = 8 mm UP and RH = 2 mm OUT. These are the necessary decentrations required to produce $4^\triangle$ UP and $2^\triangle$ out with the above lens.

Solution by protractor

Each of the above constructions can be performed on the protractor, following the rules given below.

(1) Locate the point Z on the main scale and by cursor measure the resultant prisms ZY and ZX.

(2) Calculate the decentrations necessary to produce ZY and ZX, using $c = \dfrac{P}{F}$ as before.

(3) Compound these decentrations (OP and OQ) on the main scale to find the point R.

(4) Resolve the position of R into vertical and horizontal components RV and RH.

Experiment 61
NEAR CENTRATION DISTANCE

Theory

When recording the centration distance for distance vision, we measure the distance between the centres of the pupils (PD). In near vision, however, the separation of the centres of the converging pupils is not required but, instead, the horizontal distance between the visual points measured in the spectacle plane. This distance is called the near centration distance (NCD) and is invariably less than the near inter-pupillary distance owing to the forward position of the spectacle plane.

The optical centres for near vision should be separated by the near centration distance in the absence of a prescribed prism.

An accurate measurement of the NCD usually involves the use of a special PD gauge. It can be measured by means of a simple rule provided that the ruler is held in the spectacle plane, a rough guide to which is the front plane of an empty spectacle frame. Alternatively the NCD can be calculated using assumed values for the lens—eye separation and fixation distance as outlined in exercise (1) below. It will be found that an average value for the NCD is 5 mm less than the distance PD.

Apparatus

Face measuring rule; empty spectacle frame.

Procedure

(1) Sit opposite your subject and adjust the level of your stool until your eyes are on the same level as his.

(2)   Place an empty spectacle frame on your subject's face.

(3)   Adjust the position of your head so that your left eye lies in front of your subject's nose at his conventional reading distance (about 30–40 cm, but it may vary outside these limits according to his height and posture).

(4)   Direct the subject to look at your centrally placed left eye. Your right eye should be closed.

(5)   Hold the rule against the front plane of the empty spectacle frame and adjust its position so that the zero of the scale is aligned with the temporal side of the subject's right pupil.

(6)   The rule and your own head must now be kept still.

(7)   Transfer your direction of gaze to the subject's left eye and note the position of the nasal edge of his left pupil in relation to the scale.

(8)   Record the measurement as the NCD.

(9)   Repeat the experiment for working distances of 20 cm and 50 cm.

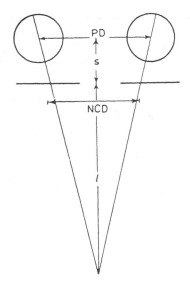

Figure 61.1

Exercises

(1)   In *Figure 61.1* the working distance measured from the spectacle plane is denoted by l, the distance from the eyes' centres of

rotation to the spectacle plane by s, the distance between the eyes'
centres of rotation by PD, and the near centration distance by NCD.

Show that $NCD = PD \times \dfrac{l}{l+s}$.

(2)   Calculate the NCD for the following values of PD. Assume that
$s = 27$ mm in each case.

PD	l = 25 cm	l = 33 cm	l = 40 cm
70 mm			
65 mm			
60 mm			
55 mm			
50 mm			

Experiment 62
LENTICULAR LENSES. MARGINAL
TOOL POWER

Theory

An application of the sag formula enables one to find the marginal tool required to produce a given aperture and edge thickness for a workshop flattened concave lenticular.

In *Figure 62.1*, it should be evident that there is only one positive curve M which will produce the desired aperture a together with a given edge substance e at the particular diameter d. A shallower curve would clearly increase the edge substance if the correct aperture were produced or, alternatively, decrease the aperture if the correct edge

Figure 62.1

substance were produced. A steeper curve than the one depicted would have the reverse effects. From the geometry of *Figure 62.1*, the following statement is easily established.

Sag M at d $-$ sag M at a $+$ sag F_1 at d $+$ e $=$ sag F_2 at a $+$ t.

M is the power of the necessary marginal tool. Rearranging this expression, we obtain

sag M at d $-$ sag M at a $=$ sag F_2 at a $-$ sag F_1 at d $-$ (e $-$ t).

This expression is easily solved if a table of lens thickness is available.

Using the tables, the right-hand side of the expression can be evaluated immediately, since all the terms should be known. The problem is then to find which surface power differs between the selected apertures a and d by the value calculated for the right-hand side of the equation.

We will assume the use of a table of sags to illustrate this direct method of solution before considering single equations.

Example

Calculate the power of the marginal tool required to produce the following workshop flattened lenticular.

Rx. − 20.00 DS diameter of uncut d = 50 mm.
F_1 = + 3.00 DS centre thickness t = 0.6 mm.
F_2 = − 23.00 DS edge thickness e = 2.6 mm.
Aperture a = 28 mm.

We begin by calculating the right-hand side of the expression

$$\text{sag } F_2 \text{ at } a - \text{sag } F_1 \text{ at } d - (e - t)$$
$$= \text{sag } 23.00 \text{ at } 28 - \text{sag } 3.00 \text{ at } 50 - (2.6 - 0.6).$$

From the sag chart we obtain immediately

$$4.82 - 1.8 - 2 = 1.02 \text{ mm}.$$

We must now find, by interpolation from the table, which surface power differs between 50 mm aperture and 28 mm aperture by 1.02 mm. An approximate value for this curve can be found as follows.

Let the above result (1.02 mm) be x, then the marginal curve

$$M \simeq \frac{4{,}000 \, x}{d^2 - a^2}$$

In this example, $M \simeq \dfrac{4{,}000 \times 1.02}{50^2 - 28^2}$ or + 2.38 D.

Inspection of the sag chart shows that the 2.50 D curve differs by 1.04 mm between apertures 50 mm and 28 mm, and this is the spectacle tool which should be used to produce the required flattening.

Equations can be derived to cope with this problem of finding the best marginal tool for any given specifications. Any exact equations, e.g.,

$$M = \frac{2,000\,(n-1)\,x}{\left\{\left[\left(\dfrac{a-d}{2}\right)^2 + x^2\right]\left[\left(\dfrac{a+d}{2}\right)^2 + x^2\right]\right\}^{\frac{1}{2}}} \qquad *$$

must be quadratic in type and extremely tedious to solve, whereas an approximate equation may not always produce the best solution.

However, the method used in the above example required the use of a sag chart and this may not always be available. An approximate expression for M is easily derived using the sag relationship

$$s = \frac{y^2 F}{1,000}$$

and substituting this linear (in terms of s and F) but approximate equation into the above statement concerning the sags of the curves.

Sag M at d − sag M at a = sag F_2 at a − sag F_1 at d − (e − t).

The substitution produces

$$\frac{\left(\dfrac{d}{2}\right)^2}{1,000} M - \frac{\left(\dfrac{a}{2}\right)^2}{1,000} M = \frac{\left(\dfrac{a}{2}\right)^2}{1,000} F_2 - \frac{\left(\dfrac{d}{2}\right)^2}{1,000} F_1 - (e - t)$$

which after transformation yields

$$M = \frac{a^2 F_2 - d^2 F_1 - 4,000\,(e - t)}{d^2 - a^2}$$

Using the values from the example,

$$M = \frac{28^2 \times 23 - 50^2 \times 3 - 4,000\,(2.6 - 0.6)}{50^2 - 28^2}$$

$$= +1.50\,D.$$

This result is 1.00 D shallower than the best solution found by the previous more exact method. If the + 1.50 D tool were used and the

---

*All dimensions are given in millimetres, the various symbols having the same meaning as in the text.

correct aperture were produced, the edge substance would be 3.2 mm and not 2.6 mm as specified.

Plano-concave and biconcave forms

So far it has been assumed that the lenticular lens is to be made up with a shallow convex base curve. This of course is not always the case, plano-conave and biconcave forms frequently being chosen.

Figure 62.2

When the front surface power is zero *(Figure 62.2a)*, sag F_1 at d is also zero and the marginal tool M, required to produce the correct aperture and edge thickness, is found from

$$M = \frac{a^2 F - 4{,}000\,(e - t)}{d^2 - a^2}$$

in which expression F is the total prescription of the lens.

In *Figure 62.2b* the front surface is a shallow concave curve and the following is easily seen.

$$\text{sag M at } d - \text{sag M at } a = \text{sag } F_2 \text{ at } a + \text{sag } F_1 \text{ at } d - (e - t)$$

$$\text{from which } M = \frac{a^2 F_2 + d^2 F_1 - 4{,}000\,(e - t)}{d^2 - a^2}$$

where, as we should expect, the term $d^2 F_1$ appears with opposite sign.

Sphero-cylindrical and toric lenticulars

When a flattened lenticular incorporates a cylindrical component, care must be taken that the correct edge thickness is obtained.

If we assume that the edge thickness specified is always the thin edge substance, then the following rules are operative:

+ base torics	take F_1 = the cross curve
∞/+ sph.-cyl.	take F_1 = the cylinder curve
∞/− sph.-cyl.	take F_1 = plano
− base torics	take F_1 = the base curve

and it can be seen that F_1 should always correspond with the most convex (or least concave) outside curve.

Oval-aperture lenticulars

The methods outlined above can be used to calculate the cylindrical or toroidal tool necessary to produce an oval-aperture lenticular of any given dimensions. Here two values for M must be calculated, one along the horizontal diameter of the aperture and one along the vertical diameter. These two values will represent the base curve and cross curve of the tool necessary to produce the aperture.

Example

Calculate the power of the plano-convex cylindrical tool required to produce the following lenticular in plano-concave form.

Rx. − 15.00 DS   oval-aperture lenticular
34 × 28 mm

centre thickness 0.6 mm, uncut diameter 48 mm round. The use of a sag chart will be assumed.

Figure 62.3

Since the horizontal aperture of the lenticular is being flattened with the axis meridian of a cylindrical tool, the edge thickness at the extremities of the horizontal diameter of the uncut, e_H, is simply sag F_2 at a_H + t or sag 15.00 at 32 + 0.6 = 3.89 + 0.6 mm or 4.49 mm. It can be seen from *Figure 62.3* that this value must also represent, in the vertical meridian of the blank, sag M_V at d + e_V. Also it will be realized from *Figure 62.3* that

sag M_V at d + e_V = sag M_V at a_V + sag F_2 at a_V + t.

Hence sag M_V at a_V = e_H − t − sag F_2 at a_V
                        = 4.49 − 0.6 − sag 15.00 at 28
                        = 3.89 − 2.93 mm
                        = 0.96 mm.

Hence M_V = + 5.00 D.

The edge thickness at the extremities of the vertical diameter of the finished uncut will be

$$e_V = e_H - \text{sag } M_V \text{ at } d = 4.49 - \text{sag } 5.00 \text{ at } 48$$
$$= 4.49 - 2.79 \text{ mm}$$
$$= 1.7 \text{ mm.}$$

The flattening tool required is $/ + 5.00 \text{ DC} \times 180$.

In the following experiment, the marginal tool power should be calculated with the aid of a table of lens thicknesses.

Apparatus

Table of lens thicknesses.

Prescriptions

(1) Rx. $- 15.00$ DS, 28 mm aperture lenticular. Form plano-concave, centre thickness 0.6 mm, edge thickness 1 mm, diameter of uncut 50 mm.

(2) Rx. $- 18.00/ + 3.00 \times 90$, 26 mm aperture lenticular. Form $\infty/ + 3.00$ DC on front surface, centre thickness 0.6 mm, thin edge 1.2 mm, diameter of uncut 46 mm.

(3) Rx. $- 12.00/ + 200 \times 180$, 34 mm aperture lenticular. Form $+ 3.00$ base toric, centre thickness 0.8 mm, thin edge 1.8 mm, diameter of uncut 54 mm.

(4) Rx. $- 14.00$ DS, 26×22 oval-aperture lenticular. Form $F_1 = + 3.00$ DS, centre thickness 0.6 mm, diameter of uncut 44 mm.

Procedure

(1) Using the table of lens thicknesses, evaluate

$$\text{sag } F_2 \text{ at } a \pm \text{sag } F_1 \text{ at } d - (e - t).$$

Sag F_1 at d should be added when F_1 is concave but subtracted when F_1 is convex. (See rules for sphero-cylindrical and toric forms to determine F_1 for astigmatic lenticulars.)

(2) Find a close value for M from

$$M = \frac{4,000 \, x}{d^2 - a^2}$$

(3)   Check the marginal tool power given in step (2), using the table of lens thicknesses. You should find

$$\text{sag M at d} - \text{sag M at a} = x.$$

Adjust the value of M if necessary.

Experiment 63
INSPECTION OF LENSES FOR
PHYSICAL DEFECTS

Theory

Finished spectacle lenses may suffer from a number of physical defects which spoil the quality or the optical performance of the lens. It is essential to be able to distinguish these defects and to relate them to their origin. We can conveniently divide the defects into two categories:

(1) Defects in the lens material.
(2) Surface defects.

There are three methods of inspecting a finished lens. The first entails looking directly into the lens material, there being a powerful source of light behind the lens. The lens should be absolutely clean and held at about 30 cm from the eye, the source of light being some distance beyond the lens. The defect is most easily seen when it lies on the line joining the source and the eye, and the lens under test must be moved around and tilted slightly so that each zone can be examined. The defects listed below which will probably be seen most easily by this method are suffixed by (T).

The second method is used for finding surface defects, the lens being held close to a source of light and the zone of the surface which is brightly illuminated by the source being examined by means of the reflected light. On moving the lens around, each zone of the surface can be examined. This method is indicated below by the suffix (R).

The third technique is known as 'shadowing'. Shadowing a lens involves holding the lens at its own focal length in front of the eye and viewing a fairly powerful source of light through the lens, a real image of the source being formed in the region of the pupil. In order to produce a real image under these conditions, the lens must be of moderate plus power, and a weak positive or negative lens would have to be combined with a plus lens of suitable power, itself free from defects. When the lens under examination is held before the source and a real image is allowed to fall on the eye, the lens will appear very bright, its whole aperture being filled with light. If the lens is slowly moved to one side, the image will move out of the pupil and at a certain point the lens will begin to darken. At this point any material or surface defects in that zone of the lens will suddenly appear. This technique is denoted by the suffix (S).

Material defects

Colour

Spectacle lens material should be completely 'white' (unless purposely tinted). Any unintended coloration usually arises from the use of impure materials in the batch. Colour may be detected by comparing the lens with a good sample on well illuminated white paper.

Strain

Strain in an unmounted lens is usually evidence of faulty annealing, the molten glass having been allowed to cool too rapidly. In a mounted lens any strain may be due to compression by the rims of the frame (or rimless screws), the lens having been overglazed. Strained glass is bi-refringent and the strain may be detected by holding the sample between two crossed polarizing filters (strain tester).

Bad metal (T)

The material of the lens should be completely free from foreign particles or undissolved batch materials.

Bubbles (T)

Bubbles are formed by the large volume of gas given off during the melt. Vigorous stirring of the glass melt should allow all the bubbles to work their way to the surface and escape. Bubbles under 0.25 mm in diameter are usually referred to as 'seeds', and a magnifying glass may be necessary to distinguish the comparative sphericity of a seed from the more irregular appearance of a speck of bad metal.

Feathers (T)

A cluster of bubbles or seeds often seen around a speck of bad metal takes on the appearance of a small white feather.

Veins (S)

A vein is a fine thread or streak of glass of slightly different refractive index from the surrounding glass. The appearance is rather like a thin empty tube running through the glass. A very fine vein is called a 'stria', while a number of pronounced veins are referred to as 'cord'.

Surface defects

Tarnish (R)

Tarnish or staining is the result of chemical changes at the lens surface. Flint glasses are especially prone to this defect, their lead content oxidizing at the surface and producing dark stains.

Crazing (R)

A defect presenting the appearance of small criss-cross cracks at the surface. It is usually caused by sudden chilling.

Hole (R)

A small pit in the lens surface which may be caused by breaking into a bubble or, more frequently, by insufficient smoothing.

Greyness (R)

Incomplete polishing.

Polishing burn (R or T)

A blister or a group of small blisters arising from insufficient lubrication of the polishing pad.

Waves (T or S)

A wave is a surface undulation, there being a change of curvature in the region of the wave. A bad wave produces a noticeable kick in a straight line under the transverse test. Special forms of waves are listed below.

Rings. – Concentric waves on a spherical surface.

Cloth marks. – A form of waviness characterized by the weave of the polishing pad on the surface.

Drag marks. – Local waves usually associated with an edge chip.

Orange peel. – A form of waviness named after its appearance.

Rounding. – A defect of figure at the edge of the lens.

Scratch (R)

An elongated penetration of the surface characterized by jagged edges.

Dig (R)

A very short scratch.

Sleek (R)

An elongated penetration of the surface without splintering.

Bruise check (R)

A surface crack or fracture due to impact on the surface of the glass.

Chips (R)

Chips usually occur at the edge of a lens, being produced either by impact or by tension applied by a spectacle frame. Shallow chips are referred to as 'flakes' or, if very small, as 'sparks'. The presence of a number of sparks left over from the glazing process is known as 'starring'.

Abuse marks (R)

This term is used to cover surface defects caused by careless handling.

In addition to the above defects, lenticular and bifocal lenses may suffer mechanical defects at their dividing lines or on their contact surfaces. In particular, with solid lenticular and bifocal lenses the dividing line should be a single line with no evidence of multiple lines or rounding over. Fused bifocals should not have any imperfections on their contact surfaces.

Apparatus

Defective lenses; strain tester; inspection chamber or shadowscope, or suitable light source and dark background; magnifying glass; lens cleaning cloth.

Procedure

(1)   Make sure that the lens is absolutely clean with no fingermarks. Check for strain.

(2)   Examine the lens material first, then each surface. Do this with and without the magnifying glass. Apply the transverse test to look for waves.

(3)   Examine the lens edge and segment dividing line or contact surface.

(4)   Record the lens number and the faults which you have found.

Experiment 64
ACCURATE TRANSPOSITION

Theory

When the thickness of a lens is taken into account, the back vertex power of the lens cannot be found merely by adding together the surface powers F_1 and F_2. The back vertex power, F'_V, is given by the expression

$$F'_V = \frac{F_1 + F_2 - t/n\, F_1 F_2}{1 - t/n\, F_1}$$

where F_1 is the power of the front surface, F_2 is the power of the back surface, t is the axial thickness of the lens, and n is the refractive index of the material from which the lens is made. With negative lenses, t is usually so small that it can be ignored and the back vertex power can be found from the sum of the surface powers. For positive lenses, however, t cannot be ignored and must be taken into account when computing the details of the lens.

A problem which arises frequently during the manufacture of positive lenses is that of finding which surface power must be used to produce a lens of given back vertex power, thickness and refractive index when the other surface power is known. The problem which arises most frequently is to find F_1 given F'_V, F_2, t and n.

TO FIND F_1

From the back vertex power formula given above, we have

$$F_1 = \frac{F'_V - F_2}{1 + t/n\, (F'_V - F_2)}$$

211

The quantity $F'_V - F_2$ is the power which would be worked on the front surface if the thickness of the lens were ignored. It is known as the nominal or uncompensated front surface power F_1N. We can write

$$F_1 = \frac{F_1N}{1 + t/n\, F_1N}$$

The actual or compensated front surface power which must be worked, F_1, is invariably lower than F_1N. It is often called the reduced front curve. The easiest method of finding F_1 is to find first its focal length in millimetres, $f_1 = \dfrac{1,000}{F_1}$, for we can then write

$$f_1 = \frac{1,000}{F_1N} + \frac{t}{n}$$

$$\text{or } f_1 = f_1N + \frac{t}{n}$$

where f_1N is the nominal focal length of the front surface in millimetres.

Examples

(1) Find the front surface power required to produce a + 6.00 DS on a − 4.00 D base curve. The axial thickness of the lens is 5 mm and it is made in glass n = 1.523. The nominal front surface power $(F'_V - F_2)$ is + 10.00 D.

$$\text{So } f_1N = \frac{1,000}{10}\,mm = 100\ mm$$

$$\frac{t}{n} = \frac{5}{1.523} = 3.28\ mm.$$

$$\text{Then } f_1 = f_1N + \frac{t}{n}$$

$$= 100 + 3.28$$

$$= 103.28\ mm$$

$$\text{and } F_1 = \frac{1,000}{f_1} = \frac{1,000}{103.28} = +9.68\ D.$$

The front surface power is therefore + 9.68 D.

(2) Find the front surface power required to produce a $+13.00$ DS with a -3.00 D base curve. Assume that $t = 8$ mm and $n = 1.523$.

$$F_1 N = F'_V - F_2 = +16.00 \text{ D}$$

$$\text{so } f_1 N = \frac{1,000}{16} \text{ mm}$$

$$= 62.5 \text{ mm}$$

$$\frac{t}{n} = \frac{8}{1.523} = 5.25 \text{ mm.}$$

Then $f_1 = f_1 N + \dfrac{t}{n}$

$$= 62.5 + 5.25$$

$$= 67.75 \text{ mm}$$

$$\text{and } F_1 = \frac{1,000}{f_1} = \frac{1,000}{67.75} = +14.76 \text{ D.}$$

The front surface power is therefore $+14.76$ D.

(3) It is required to produce the lens $+8.00/+4.00 \times 90$ in toric form with a -3.00 D base curve. The lens is to be 6 mm thick and made in glass $n = 1.523$. Find the front surface power.

The form of the lens is $\dfrac{+15.00 \text{ DS (nominal)}}{-3.00 \text{ DC} \times 90/-7.00 \text{ DC} \times 180}$

$$\text{so } F_1 N = +15.00 \text{ D}$$

$$f_1 N = \frac{1,000}{15} = 66.67 \text{ mm}$$

$$\frac{t}{n} = \frac{6}{1.523} = 3.94 \text{ mm.}$$

Then $f_1 = f_1 N + \dfrac{t}{n}$

$$= 66.67 + 3.94$$

$$= 70.61 \text{ mm}$$

$$\text{and } F_1 = \frac{1,000}{70.61} = +14.16 \text{ D.}$$

The advantages of using a minus base toric form for these high powered lenses is shown in this last example. It is seen that it is only necessary to compensate the spherical curve. If the above lens had been made with a sphere curve on the back surface, it would have been necessary to compensate both the base curve and the cross curve of the convex toroidal surface as shown by the following example.

(4) It is required to produce the lens $+ 8.00/ + 4.00 \times 90$ in toric form with a $- 3.00$ D sphere curve. Using $t = 6$ mm and $n = 1.523$, find the surface powers required on the toric surface.

The form of the lens is $\dfrac{+ 11.00 \text{ DC} \times 180/ + 15.00 \text{ DC} \times 90}{- 3.00 \text{ DS}}$

The curves on the toroidal surface are of course the nominal front surface powers. It is necessary to compensate both of these. The cross curve $+ 15.00$ DC (nominal), however, has already been compensated in the last example. We saw there that a $+ 15.00$ D curve at 6 mm thickness becomes $+ 14.16$ D; Compensating the base curve meridian, we find

$$f_1 N = 90.91 \text{ mm}$$

$$f_1 = 90.97 + 3.94$$

$$= 94.91 \text{ mm}$$

$$\text{and } F_1 = + 10.54 \text{ D.}$$

The actual surface powers must therefore be

$$\frac{+ 10.54 \text{ DC} \times 180/ + 14.16 \text{ DC} \times 90}{- 3.00 \text{ DS}}$$

The difference between the compensated and uncompensated front surface powers is called the front surface vertex power allowance VPA_1.

We have $VPA_1 = F_1 - F_1 N$.

Since $F_1 = \dfrac{F_1 N}{1 + t/n \, F_1 N}$

we can write $VPA_1 = \dfrac{- t/n \, F_1 N^2}{1 + t/n \, F_1 N}$ (t in metres).

The vertex power allowance for example (1) above is

$$VPA_1 = \frac{- 0.00328 \times 10^2}{1 + 0.00328 \times 10}$$

$$= \frac{-0.328}{1.0328}$$

$$= -0.32 \text{ D.}$$

and the compensated front surface power is $+ 9.68$ D as before.

It will be left as an exercise for the student to show that the vertex power allowances for examples (2) to (4) are:

(2) $- 1.24$ D.
(3) $- 0.84$ D.
(4) $- 0.46$ D (base curve) $- 0.84$ D (cross curve).

TO FIND F_2

When it is required to compensate the back surface of the lens, the expression for F_2 cannot be put into such a simple and convenient form in terms of its focal length. From the back vertex power formula we have

$$F_2 = F'_V - \frac{F_1}{1 - t/n\, F_1}$$

$$= \frac{F'_V - t/n\, F_1\, F'_V - F_1}{1 - t/n\, F_1}$$

$$= \frac{F_2 N - t/n\, F_1\, (F_1 + F_2 N)}{1 - t/n\, F_1}$$

where $F_2 N$ is the nominal or uncompensated back surface power $F'_V - F_1$.

If we put this straight into the form which gives the back surface vertex power allowance, $VPA_2 = F_2 - F_2 N$, the expression reduces finally to

$$VPA_2 = \frac{- t/n\, F_1{}^2}{1 - t/n\, F_1}$$

This should be compared with the expression for VPA_1.

Examples

(1) Find the back surface power required to produce a $+ 6.00$ D lens with a $+ 10.00$ D front surface power. The axial thickness of the lens is 5 mm and it is made in glass $n = 1.523$.

$$VPA_2 = \frac{-t/n\ F_1{}^2}{1 - t/n\ F_1}$$

$$= \frac{-0.00328 \times 10^2}{1 - 0.00328 \times 10}$$

$$= \frac{-0.328}{0.9672}$$

$$= -0.34\ D.$$

$$F_2 = VPA_2 + F_2N$$

$$= -0.34 - 4$$

$$= -4.34\ D.$$

(2) Find the back surface power required to produce a + 13.00 DS with a + 16.00 D front surface power. Assume that t = 8 mm and n = 1.523.

$$VPA_2 = \frac{-0.00525 \times 16^2}{1 - 0.00525 \times 16}$$

$$= \frac{-1.344}{0.916}$$

$$= -1.47\ D.$$

$$F_2 = VPA_2 + F_2N$$

$$= -1.47 - 3$$

$$= -4.47\ D.$$

(3) It is required to produce the lens + 8.00/+ 4.00 × 90 in toric form with a + 15.00 D sphere curve. The lens is to be 8 mm thick and made in glass n = 1.523. Find the powers required on the toroidal surface.

The form of the lens is $\dfrac{+\ 15.00\ DS}{-\ 3.00\ DC \times 90/-\ 7.00\ DC \times 180}$

the toroidal surface powers being the nominal curves. Each meridian must be considered separately, but the vertex power allowance for each curve on the toroidal surface is the same.

$$VPA_2 = \frac{-0.00525 \times 15^2}{1 - 0.00525 \times 15}$$

$$= \frac{-1.181}{0.9213}$$

$$= -1.28 \text{ D.}$$

$$F_2 \text{ (base)} = VPA_2 + F_2 N \text{ (base)}$$

$$= -1.28 - 3$$

$$= -4.28 \text{ D.}$$

$$F_2 \text{ (cross)} = VPA_2 + F_2 N \text{ (cross)}$$

$$= -1.28 - 7$$

$$= -8.28 \text{ D.}$$

The actual surface powers are therefore

$$\frac{+15.00 \text{ DS}}{-4.28 \text{ DC} \times 90 / -8.28 \text{ DC} \times 180}$$

Experiment 65
INSPECTION OF SPECIAL
SPECTACLE LENSES

Theory

This experiment is designed to facilitate the recognition of different types of spectacle lenses. In addition, it should draw your attention to the detailed information required to familiarize yourself with the various lens types which are available.

Special spectacle lenses will be classified into six main groups:

(1)   Lenses for myopia.
(2)   Lenses for aphakia.
(3)   Lenses for anisometropia.
(4)   Bifocal lenses.
(5)   Multifocal lenses.
(6)   Tinted and protective lenses.

Tinted lenses are dealt with in Experiment 68, and you should consider here only lenses which offer mechanical protection in group (6).

Much of the detailed information which you require will be found in *Lens Forms,* and you should refer to this booklet as necessary.

You should pay special attention to the following general items which you are required to record:

(1)   Media in which the lens can be made.
(2)   Available forms (standard base curves).
(3)   Available aperture or segment sizes.
(4)   Maximum blank size.
(5)   Standard tints in which the lens can be made.
(6)   Power range, if limited by manufacturer.

In addition, you should consider the following.

Single vision lenses

(1) What advantage does the lens type have over full aperture lenses?

(2) Is the edge thickness sufficient to warrant a special edging technique?

(3) What will be the appearance of the wearer's eyes behind a pair of these lenses?

(4) If the lenses are to be used for distance vision, is the field of view adequate?

Bifocal lenses

(1) Does the lens type offer control over the prismatic effect at the near visual point?

(2) What is the jump exerted by the segment at its dividing line?

(3) Is the chromatism in the near visual zone excessive?

(4) Is the dividing line relatively inconspicuous?

(5) Is the bifocal permanent?

(6) Can useful distance vision be obtained beneath the reading area?

(7) Is the near field of view adequate?

Multifocal lenses

(1) What ranges of vision are obtainable through the separate zones? If a trifocal design, can the IP/RP ratio be varied?

(2) What is the position of the intermediate zone?

(3) If the lens is a varifocal, what is the approximate area of useful vision?

Protective lenses

(1) Is the lens more break-resistant than ordinary glass?

(2) What size, power and thickness restrictions are imposed?

(3) When the lens is broken, what type of fragmentation is obtained?

Apparatus

Sets of special lenses, lens measure, *Lens Form* booklet, ruler.

Procedure

(1) Record the correct name of the lens.
(2) Sketch frontal and cross-sectional views of the lens.
(3) State the medium from which the lens is made.
(4) State any other media in which the lens is available.
(5) Record the base curve (or DP curve or other defining curve) of the lens. Do any other forms exist?
(6) Record any lenticular aperture dimension or segment diameter or size.
(7) Record the maximum blank size.
(8) Record the power range in which the lens is available.
(9) State what limitations exist with regard to tints.
(10) Answer the questions posed under the general headings above.

Use a whole page of your answer sheets for each lens form.

Experiment 66
TO DETERMINE THE TRANSMISSION FACTORS OF OPHTHALMIC TINTED LENSES

Theory

A tinted lens reduces the total amount of light reaching the eye, but its transmission generally varies according to the wavelength of the light. In this experiment, the luminous transmission factor or integrated visible transmission factor is determined. This can be defined as the ratio of the luminous flux transmitted by a lens to that which it receives.

Apparatus

Joly wax photometer; Bunsen grease spot photometer; Lummer–Brodhun photometer; optical bench; two sources; two diaphragms about 40 mm in diameter; Crookes B_1 and B_2 glasses.

Procedure

Set up the apparatus as shown in *Figure 66.1,* first of all without the tinted glass in position, and determine the photometric balance.

Then it can be shown that $\dfrac{I_1}{d_1{}^2} = \dfrac{I_2}{d_2{}^2}$.

I_1 and I_2 are the luminous intensities or candle powers of the sources.

Hence $I_1 = kI_2$ where $k = \dfrac{d_1{}^2}{d_2{}^2}$.

Place the tinted glass in position and determine the new photometric balance for distances d_3 and d_4.

Then $\dfrac{t.I_1}{d_3{}^2} = \dfrac{I_2}{d_4{}^2}$ where t = transmission factor.

$$t = \frac{I_2}{I_1} \cdot \frac{d_3{}^2}{d_4{}^2} = \frac{1}{k}\left(\frac{d_3}{d_4}\right)^2$$

t can be expressed as a percentage or as a decimal.

Another way of expressing the transmission factor is by the concept of optical density where

$$\text{optical density } D = \log_{10}\frac{1}{t} \text{ (t as a decimal).}$$

Determine t and D for the two glasses given individually and with the two placed in series.

Note that $t_{12} = t_1 . t_2$
$$D_{12} = D_1 + D_2.$$

Repeat the experiment for the other photometer heads provided. Comment on any differences in the results.

Figure 66.1. For clarity the components have been drawn separately, but theoretically the lamp, diaphragm and tint should lie in the same plane, distance d_1 from the photometer head. The second lamp and the diaphragm are likewise distance d_2 away

Remember that the experiment should be performed in as complete darkness as possible and reflecting surfaces such as notebooks should be kept away from the lights.

Example

On an optical bench a photometric balance is obtained when the photometer head is 100 cm from either source. A tinted lens which has

222

a transmission factor of $(64/81)$ is placed before one source. What is the position of the photometer for the new photometric balance?

Another tinted lens with a transmission factor of $(81/100)$ is placed in contact with the tinted lens. How far must the photometer be moved and in which direction to obtain a photometric balance? What is the transmission factor of the composite tinted lens?

Show that the optical density of the composite tinted lens is the sum of the optical densities of each lens.

Answer

Refer to *Figure 66.1*.

The photometer head is midway between the two sources.

I_1 and I_2 are 200 cm apart.

$$\therefore d_1 = d_2 = 100 \text{ cm.}$$

Hence $\dfrac{I_1}{100^2} = \dfrac{I_2}{100^2}$

$$\therefore I_1 = I_2 \text{ and } k = 1.$$

(1) Tinted glass in position $\dfrac{t_1 I_1}{d_3{}^2} = \dfrac{I_2}{d_4{}^2}$

$t_1 = \dfrac{81}{100}, I_1 = I_2 \text{ and } d_3 = (200 - d_4)$

$$\therefore \frac{81}{100} \times \frac{11}{(200 - d_4)^2} = \frac{1}{d_4{}^2}$$

Take square roots each side, $\dfrac{9}{10} \times \dfrac{1}{(200 - d_4)} = \dfrac{1}{d_4}$

Hence $d_4 = 105.3$ cm.

The photometer head is moved towards the source masked by the tinted lens.

(2) Composite tinted lens has a transmission factor $t = t_1 \times t_2$

where $t_1 = \dfrac{81}{100}, \ t_2 = \dfrac{64}{81}, \ \therefore t = \dfrac{64}{100}$

For photometric balance, $t \times \dfrac{I_1}{d'_3{}^2} = \dfrac{I_2}{d'_4{}^2}$ where d'_3 and d'_4 are the new distances.

$$t = \frac{64}{100}, \quad I_1 = I_2, \text{ and } d'_3 = (200 - d'_4).$$

$$\therefore \frac{64}{100} \times \frac{1}{(200 - d'_4)^2} = \frac{1}{d'_4{}^2}$$

Taking square roots each side, $\dfrac{8}{10} \cdot \dfrac{1}{(200 - d'_4)} = \dfrac{1}{d'_4}$

and $d'_4 = 111.1$ cm, therefore the photometer head must be moved towards the composite tinted lens a distance $111.1 - 105.3 = 5.8$ cm.

Optical density D_1 of first tinted lens is given by $\log_{10} \dfrac{1}{t}$,

$$\text{hence } D_1 = \log_{10} \frac{1}{0.81}$$

$$= \log_{10} 1.235$$

$$= 0.0915.$$

$$D_2 = \log_{10} \frac{1}{64/81}$$

$$= \log_{10} 1.265$$

$$= 0.1023.$$

Optical density D of the first and second tinted lenses in contact is:

$$D = \log_{10} \frac{1}{64/100}$$

$$= \log_{10} 1.563$$

$$= 0.1938.$$

$D_1 + D_2 = 0.1938$, the optical density D.

Experiment 67
THE POCKET SPECTROSCOPE

Theory

This simple piece of apparatus enables us to identify various spectrum sources or filters. The instrument consists of a train of five prisms which produce a brilliant spectrum dispersed through $10°$ of arc. There is an adjustable slit and a focusing drawtube. Do not close the jaws completely or the instrument will be damaged.

Apparatus

Pocket spectroscope; sets of filters; sources; daylight source if available; tinted ophthalmic lenses with transmission charts.

Procedure

Look through the spectroscope at a daylight source or at an incandescent source. Alter the width of the slit and/or adjust the focusing drawtube until a well-defined spectrum is observed. Sketch this spectrum. Place one of the filters from the numbered set in front of the spectroscope; observe and sketch the resultant spectrum. Repeat for each filter in turn, sketching the spectra to scale one below the other.

Now select two of the filters, place them together in contact and sketch the resultant spectrum. Compare this with the spectrum due to each filter alone. Give your conclusions and observations. Repeat with other pairs of filters.

From the above results, comment on the quality of the filters. Repeat the experiment with tinted ophthalmic lenses. Compare the resultant spectrum with the relevant transmission chart.

Exercise

Give an example of the use of a tinted ophthalmic lens.

Experiment 68
TINTED SPECTACLE LENSES

Theory

When protection is required for the eyes against undesirable radiant energy, it can be provided in the form of a tinted lens or filter. Filters modify the intensity and spectral distribution of the radiant energy which they transmit. The modification may result from absorption by the filter or from reflection from one specially treated surface.

Protection is usually required against radiations within and just outside the visible spectrum. The important wavebands are as follows.

1. Glare within the visible waveband (390 nm → 760 nm approx.)

Any brightness within the visible spectrum which produces visual discomfort. Glare can usually be attributed to levels of illumination in excess of those to which the subject is normally accustomed. Neutral filters (*see below*) or filters which absorb or reflect strongly in the middle of the visible spectrum are usually employed.

2. Ultra-violet radiation (10 nm → 390 nm approx.)

Exposure usually arises from the reflection of the sun's energy from expanses of sand, sea, snow or concrete road. It also arises in industrial occupations such as welding, from arc lamps in cinema and photographic studios, or from physiotherapy. Ultra-violet is particularly insidious because it does not directly stimulate the sensory nervous system and there is no apparent warning of the hazard.

Filters which obstruct ultra-violet radiation below 360 nm are employed. The absorptive filters generally contain cerium oxide and are pink in colour.

3. Infra-red radiation (760 nm → 500,000 nm approx.)

Infra-red radiation is invariably accompanied by a sensation of warmth. Exposure usually arises from industrial pursuits such as furnace working. Glass workers are typically subject to this hazard. Staring hard at the sun may provoke lesions in the macula. Fair-skinned people whose environment changes to a tropical climate may require protection against infra-red radiation.

Filters which obstruct radiation above 760 nm are employed. The absorptive filters generally contain ferrous oxide and are green in colour.

Apart from providing protection against the above groups of radiation, filters may also be required for the following purposes.

4. Heat-absorbing filters

These absorb infra-red radiation without absorbing strongly in the visible spectrum. They are usually pale blue-green in colour, with their peak transmission at about 500 nm.

5. Neutral grey filters

These filters do not distort colour values since their transmission is almost constant throughout the visible spectrum. They are usually a blue-grey colour.

6. Yellow absorbing filters

Of all colours, yellow possesses the highest luminosity and has the greatest effect in causing dazzle. Filters which strongly absorb the yellow region of the spectrum therefore decrease dazzle and, at the same time, increase the contrast between the red and blue ends of the visible spectrum.

7. Contrast filters

These absorb all radiation below 450 nm, their transmission curves then rising to level out at about 525 nm. The absorptive variety

227

generally contain cadmium, or chromium and are bright yellow in colour. Because they absorb the blue end of the visible spectrum, they enhance the contrast between light and dark, thereby making the boundary between light and dark areas easier to distinguish.

8. Photochromic filters

These contain microscopic crystals of silver halides which are decomposed by long wave ultra-violet into silver and halogen, darkening the glass. The halogen is held within the glass matrix and is available for recombination with the silver when the exciting source is removed, allowing the glass to regain its original colourless state. The process is speediest at low temperatures.

9. Polarizing filters

In addition to absorbing unwanted radiation, these filters absorb plane polarized light, the latter usually occurring by reflection. Polarizing filters allow objects which may appear diffused by reflected glare to be seen more closely. The polarizing axis of such a filter is normally mounted vertically before an eye.

The following mechanical definitions are used in relation to tinted lenses to describe various forms of filters and, in particular, how the tint is imparted to the lens.

A. Solid tint

The material itself is tinted throughout and the depth of tint varies with the thickness of the material. (In high power lenses, this results in a variation of tint from centre to edge.) Such filters absorb unwanted radiation.

B. Deposited tint

A chemical substance, frequently a metal or a metallic compound, is deposited upon one surface of a glass lens in a high vacuum. These tints are even in depth (equitint). Such filters reflect unwanted radiation.

C. Equitint

Any filter which displays an even depth of tint. Deposited tints are equitints. An equitint filter can also be produced by unisealing or flashing (fusing) a parallel layer of tinted material to a white lens. With plastics media, the parallel layer may be polymerized to a white plastics lens or a white lens may be dyed, the dye penetrating to an even depth throughout the plastics material.

D. Gradutint

A filter which displays a variation in tint across its face. The term is usually reserved for a filter where the gradation is deliberate, e.g., from dark at the top to white at the bottom. Gradutints may be obtained either by employing a wedged-shaped solid tint unisealed to a white base or by deposition.

In the following experiment, various types of filters are to be examined, together with their transmission curves, and the filters classified into one of the above groups. A transmission curve is a graph of the spectral transmission factor, $T\lambda$, plotted against a series of wavelengths. The spectral transmission factor, STF, is the ratio of the radiant energy transmitted by a lens to the radiant energy incident upon the lens for the specified wavelength λ.

The luminous transmission factor, LTF, is the ratio of the luminous flux transmitted by the lens to that which it receives. LTF expresses the overall effect of a filter upon an eye. (Very approximately, the LTF of a given filter corresponds with the STF at about 580 nm.)

B.S.2738, *Spectacle Lenses,* gives the following statement with reference to tinted lenses.

Tinted lenses shall not depart significantly in transmission characteristics from the manufacturer's or supplier's published figures for the particular material. Tinted material shall not be used for lenses unless the following characteristics of the material have been made freely available:

(a)   Transmission curves for a specimen 2 mm thick over the range 300 to 1,000 nm.

(b)   The luminous transmission factor for C.I.E. Standard Illuminant C at 2 mm and at least one other stated thickness of material.

(c)   When special heat absorbing properties are claimed for the material, the transmission curve for a specimen 2 mm thick over the range 1,000 to 4,000 nm and the transmission factor of a specimen 2 mm thick for total radiation (total heat) as measured by the method defined in B.S.679.

(In B.S.679, *Protective Filters for Welding and Other Industrial Occupations*, total radiation is defined as the radiation of all wavelengths of a gas-filled tungsten filament lamp modified by two reflections at aluminized mirrors and transmission by a slab of crystalline quartz 4 mm thick.)

Apparatus

Sets of filters together with their transmission curves and data.

Procedure

(1)   Ensure that you have the transmission data for the filter which you are examining.

(2)   Record the name and shade of the filter and draw a rough sketch of its transmission curve between 300 and 1,000 mm.

(3)   Record the following STF: T_{350}, T_{550}, $T_{1,000}$. Circle these points on your transmission curve.

(4)   Record the LTF and compare it with the STF at 580 mm.

(5)   State the type of filter and its transmission group, using the code letters and numbers employed above. For example, A6 would refer to a solid tint yellow absorbing filter.

(6)   Describe the colour of the filter and the visual impression you obtain when looking through it, i.e., colour distortion, whether the scene appears cloudy or sunny, etc.

Use a whole page of your answer sheets for each filter.

Experiment 69
INTERPRETATION OF PRESCRIPTIONS

Theory

This experiment involves the examination of prescriptions presented by patients for possible errors and unusual features. Also the most suitable type of lens must be selected and the complete lens specification written out as it would be ordered from the prescription house.

The prescription analysis should be approached in the following manner.

Type of prescription

Try to assess the implications of the prescription. Is it different from the patient's previous prescription? Has there been a radical change? Will the patient have any difficulty in getting used to the new prescription? Knowledge of the visual acuity will help in answering these questions.

Unusual prescriptions and omissions

Is the prescription complete? Are all the signs and axis directions shown? Are the prism base directions in opposition to one another? Are the reading additions the same in each eye? Are the cylinder powers and axis directions the same for distance and near vision?

These unusual features or omissions may require confirmation from the prescriber. A prescription should only be altered by the prescriber. A frequent omission is the vertex distance on moderate or high powered prescriptions. (The British Standard suggests that powers over ± 5.00 D should include the vertex distance.) There is little point in querying the vertex distance if it has not been considered. Strictly the patient should return to the prescriber.

Possible lens types

Consult the *Lens Forms* booklet. Decide upon the various types of lens which would be suitable for the prescription. High powered lenses may require to be made in lenticular form to reduce their weight and thickness. If full aperture lenses are to be used, what is likely to be the maximum thickness of the lens? If the lenses are to be used for both distance and near vision, analyse the centration in the near visual zone. Does the vertical relative prismatic effect exceed $1^\triangle$? Is the horizontal relative prismatic effect of large amount? Pay particular attention to the effect of the cylinder during this analysis.

If the prescription requires bifocal lenses, the following details must also be considered.

Mechanical details of lenses
Segments, permanent and inconspicuous
Optical performance of reading portion
Amount of prismatic effect in near visual zones
Jump
Differential prismatic effect in near visual zones and extent of near field of view.

Final lens choice

The final solution which you offer should take into account the vocational use of the lenses and the type and form of lens which the subject has previously worn.

Apparatus

Sets of prescriptions; *Lens Form* booklet; prescription order form.

Procedure

(1) Read each prescription through twice in order to assess the implications of the prescription and to verify that it is complete (*see* section above on unusual prescriptions and omissions).

(2) Consult the *Lens Form* booklet for the various types of lenses and media suitable for the prescription.

(3)   If bifocal lenses are prescribed, compute the prismatic effects which would occur at the near visual points.

(4)   Determine the type and form of lens which you consider most suitable for the prescription and the vocation of the patient.

(5)   Write a complete order for the lenses on the prescription order form as though they were being ordered from a prescription house. Make sure that your order is complete and free from ambiguity.

Experiment 70
THE SILWING SAGOMETER

Theory

The Silwing sagometer is a very accurate form of lens measure which may be used to determine the surface power of a lens or surfacing tool to within 0.01 D.

Whereas an ordinary lens measure records surface powers directly, the sagometer records only the sag of a curve, but by comparing the sag of an unknown curve with that of a known master curve the difference in power between the two curves may be deduced and hence the power of the unknown curve determined. The instrument is sometimes referred to as a *comparison spherometer*.

The instrument

The small red central dial records the movement of the centre leg in millimetres and the large black outer dial subdivides each millimetre step into 100 parts. The movement of the centre leg may therefore be read with ease to an accuracy of 0.01 mm.

The yoke of the instrument which carries the fixed outer legs is adjustable by loosening the screw at the rear of the yoke. In general the yoke must be moved upward in order to measure concave curves and downward in order to measure convex curves. The feet of the three legs are ball-pointed to minimize wear and prevent damage to the surface under test. Because the yoke is adjustable and the ball-pointed feet are unlikely to become worn, the accuracy of the instrument is maintained for much longer periods than that of an ordinary lens measure. In particular, any wear of the delicate internal mechanism can be ignored, since the wear is reflected on both the master curve and the curve under test at the time of use. However, the distance between the two fixed outer legs is critical and care must be taken never to exert pressure on these legs.

The master curves

The master curves provided are (very nearly):

Plano

±3.00	±12.00
±6.00	±15.00
±9.00	±18.00

The tables are calibrated for the same refractive index as the medium from which the master lenses are made (in this case 1.523).

You should avoid touching the curved surfaces themselves and *never* place a plus curve face down on the bench. Do not mate the curves. Replace the master curves in their correct positions in the box as soon as they have been measured.

The tables

Two separate tables are provided, one for convex (plus) curves and the other for concave (minus) curves.

The difference in surface power between the master curve and the unknown curve may be read directly from the tables. The first column in the tables gives the difference in gauge divisions obtained from the readings taken on the two curves. It is this value that the sagometer is used to determine. These differences are expressed in hundredths of a millimetre (i.e., 36 means 36 hundredths or 0.36 mm). When the difference has been found, the main body of the tables can be consulted to discover the difference in dioptres between the actual power of the master curve and the power of the curve under test.

Procedure

(1) Use a lens measure to provide an approximate value of the power of the curve under test.

(2) Select the master curve nearest to this and adjust the yoke of the sagometer to enable a reading to be taken on this master curve. Make sure that the adjustable yoke screw is tight, but do not overtighten it. Record the reading given on the master curve.

235

(3) Without adjusting the yoke, take a reading on the curve under test. Record this reading.

(4) Subtract the lesser reading from the greater to obtain the difference between the sags of the two curves.

(5) Using the correct set of tables, look down the first column until you find the difference recorded in step (4). Read horizontally against this difference, in the column headed by the power nearest to that of the master curve, the difference between the power of the curve under test and the master curve. Add or subtract *(see below)* this amount to the power *marked on the master curve itself* to obtain the true power of the curve under test.

Convex (plus) curve under test

If the reading on this curve is greater than that on the master curve, the curve under test is stronger (more plus) than the master curve. The difference should be added.

If the reading on the curve under test is less than that on the master curve, the curve under test is weaker (less plus) than the master curve. The difference should be subtracted.

Concave (minus) curve under test

If the reading on this curve is greater than that on the master curve, the curve under test is weaker (less minus) than the master curve. The difference should be numerically subtracted.

If the reading on the curve under test is less than that on the master curve, the curve under test is stronger (more minus) than the master curve. The difference should be numerically added.

Example

(1) Lens measure reading on unknown curve = − 8.25.

(2) Select master curve − 8.97 (i.e., approximately − 9.00). Sagometer reading on this master curve = 2.16 (i.e., 2 + on red scale, 16 on black scale).

(3) Sagometer reading on unknown curve = 2.50 (2 + on red scale, 50 on black scale).

(4) Difference = 34/100 (greater).

(5) From tables read against 34 (first column) and under − 9.00; difference in power = 0.75.

Since the reading on the unknown curve is greater, the power of the curve under test is − (8.97 − 0.75) = − 8.22 D.

Note. – It is important that the sagometer be placed perpendicularly to the curve being measured in order to obtain a true reading. You can ensure that the instrument is correctly positioned by gently rocking it over the surface in a direction at right angles to the line of the three legs and watching the movement of the pointer. With a convex (plus) curve you should record the minimum reading and with a concave (minus) curve the maximum reading obtained.

Compilation of the tables

If we are given a function $y = f(x)$, then

$$\lim_{\delta x \to 0} \left(\frac{\delta y}{\delta x} \right) = \frac{dy}{dx}.$$

If δy is considered as the very small error in y introduced by a very small error δx in x, we can write approximately

$$\delta y = \frac{dy}{dx} . \delta x.$$

The tables give the difference (or error) in surface power δF when the difference in sag, δs, is known, and from the foregoing,

$$\delta F = \frac{dF}{ds} . \delta s.$$

We require the differential coefficient $\frac{dF}{ds}$. Employing the well-known relationships

$$F = \frac{(n-1)}{r} \qquad \dots (1)$$

$$\text{and } r = \frac{y^2 + s^2}{2s} \qquad \dots (2)$$

we obtain by differentiation

$$\frac{dF}{dr} = \frac{-(n-1)}{r^2}$$

$$\text{and } \frac{dr}{ds} = \frac{s-r}{s}.$$

Since $\dfrac{dF}{dr} \times \dfrac{dr}{ds} = \dfrac{dF}{ds}$, we find

$$\frac{dF}{ds} = \frac{(r-s)(n-1)}{sr^2}$$

or introducing equation (1),

$$\frac{dF}{ds} = \frac{[(n-1)-sF]\ F}{(n-1)\ s}$$

and finally $\delta F = \dfrac{[(n-1)-sF]\ F}{(n-1)\ s} \cdot \delta s.$

For glass of refractive index 1.523 and assuming s to be substituted in millimetres,

$$\delta F = \frac{(523 - sF)\ F}{523s} \cdot \delta s \qquad \ldots (3)$$

The quantity s is the sag of the curve F at the diameter $2y'$ between the points of contact of the ball-pointed feet of the outer legs of the sagometer. It can be seen from *Figure 70.1* that the distance $2y'$ is not

Figure 70.1

the same as the distance between the centres of the balls; this latter distance we will denote by $2y$.

From the geometry of *Figure 70.1* we can easily deduce that

$$y' = \frac{yr}{r \pm r_B} \qquad \ldots (4)$$

238

r is the radius of curvature of the surface under test and r_B is the radius of curvature of the ball-pointed feet. The denominator of this expression for y' would be $r + r_B$ for convex surfaces, as depicted in *Figure 70.1*, or $r - r_B$ for concave surfaces.

An example will help to demonstrate the numerical compilation of the tables. We will choose the master curve + 12.00 D. The distance between the centres of the outer ball-pointed feet is 40 mm (i.e., y = 20 mm) and the radii of curvature of the balls themselves, r_B, is 1.6 mm. The radius of curvature of the 12.00 D surface is found by equation (1) to be 523/12 mm or 43.58 mm.

From equation (4),

$$y' = \frac{20 \times 43.58}{43.58 + 1.6} = 19.29 \text{ mm.}$$

The diameter of the chord of contact of the outer feet on the +12.00 D surface is $2y' = 38.58$ mm.

The quantity s, required for the solution of equation (3), is sag 12.00 at 38.58 mm, and from the transposed form of equation (2), $s = r - \sqrt{(r^2 - y^2)}$, we find s = 4.50 mm.

Finally, solving equation (3) we have

$$\delta F = \frac{(523 - 4.5 \times 12)\,12}{523 \times 4.5}.\,\delta s$$

or $\delta F = 2.39 . \delta s$.

Expressing the difference in gauge divisions, δs, in hundredths of a millimetre we have

$$\delta F = 0.0239 . \delta s.$$

The column headed + 12.00 D in the tables is compiled from this relation.

Experiment 71
THE ASTIGMATIC BEAM

EXPERIMENT 71A — IMAGE FORMATION BY ASTIGMATIC LENSES

Theory

Figure 71.1 shows arc ABD which is part of a circle whose centre is at C. If arc ABD is rotated about the point C, a spherical surface will be generated, but if it is rotated about any other point on the axis lying through points B and C, a toroidal surface will be generated. When rotated about the point E, the arc will form a barrel surface, but when it is rotated about the point F, a capstan surface will be formed. If arc ABD is replaced by a straight line, then a plano-cylindrical surface will be generated.

Figure 71.2 shows light from a point source B on the optical axis incident on a lens one surface of which is toroidal or plano-cylindrical, the other surface being spherical. The refracted beam does not come to a point focus but passes through two perpendicular lines at B'_H and B'_V. A pencil of light with this property is called an astigmatic beam.

The astigmatic pencil shown in *Figure 71.2* has been formed by a sphero-cylindrical or toric lens of positive focal power whose principal meridians are vertical and horizontal, the horizontal meridian having the greater focal power.

Light passing through the narrow vertical element VOV' is converged to the point B'_V on the axis of the lens; for elements parallel to VOV', light is focused at points on a horizontal line passing through B'_V, so that a horizontal line focus is formed.

240

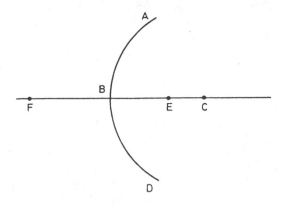

Figure 71.1. Arc ABD is part of a circle whose centre is at C. If arc ABD is rotated about any point on the axis other than C, a toroidal surface is generated

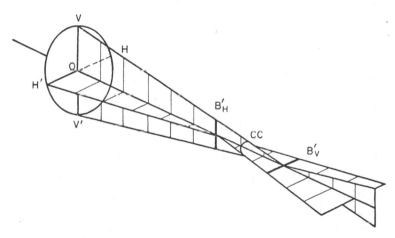

Figure 71.2. The refracted beam has initially a circular cross section which becomes elliptical, major axis vertical. At positions B'_H and CC the cross sections are a vertical line and a circle respectively. The cross section again becomes elliptical with major axis horizontal, and at B'_V a horizontal line focus is formed

Light passing through the narrow horizontal element HOH' is focused at the point B'_H on the axis of the lens. Each of the other horizontal elements of the lens brings the light to a point focus on a vertical line through B'_H, so that a vertical line focus is formed.

If the lens is circular, then at the lens the refracted beam will have a circular cross section. Between the points O and B'_H the cross section of the astigmatic beam changes from a circle to an ellipse whose major axis is vertical, to become a vertical line at B'_H.

The cross section then becomes circular at CC, after which it becomes an ellipse whose major axis is horizontal, and at B'_V it becomes a horizontal straight line. The length of the line foci and the diameter of the circular cross section at CC depend on the focal power of the lens and its diameter. The circular cross section at CC is known as the disc of least confusion.

Figure 71.3 is another version of *Figure 71.2*. The section of the astigmatic beam in the horizontal meridian is shown in full lines and the

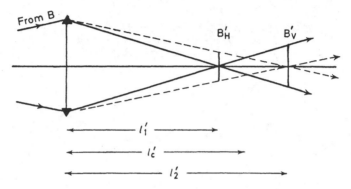

Figure 71.3. The vertical and horizontal line foci are distant l'_1 and l'_2 from the lens respectively; l'_c is the distance between the lens and the disc of least confusion

section in the vertical meridian in broken lines. A luminous point object B on the axis is imaged by the lens as an astigmatic beam. B is distant l from the lens.

Let $2y$ = diameter of lens
   l'_1 = distance of vertical line focus
   l'_c = distance of circle of least confusion
   l'_2 = distance of horizontal line focus.

Then if distances l and $2y$ are known, l'_1 and l'_2 can be determined by applying the conjugate foci relationship to each meridian.

From *Figure 71.3*,

$$\frac{\text{length of vertical line focus}}{2y} = \frac{l'_2 - l'_1}{l'_2}$$

$$\text{or length of vertical line focus} = 2y \left(\frac{L'_1 - L'_2}{L'_1} \right) \quad \ldots (1)$$

$$\text{Likewise length of horizontal line focus} = 2y \left(\frac{l'_2 - l'_1}{l'_1} \right)$$

$$= 2y \left(\frac{L'_1 - L'_2}{L'_2} \right) \quad \ldots (2)$$

Let the circle of least confusion have diameter z.

$$\text{Then } \frac{z}{2y} = \frac{l'_c - l'_1}{l'_1} = \frac{l'_2 - l'_c}{l'_2} \quad \ldots (3)$$

$$\text{Hence } l'_2 (l'_c - l'_1) = l'_1 (l'_2 - l'_c)$$

$$\text{which gives } l'_c = \frac{2l'_1 l'_2}{l'_1 + l'_2} \quad \ldots (4)$$

$$\text{From equations (3) and (4), } z = 2y \left(\frac{L'_1 - L'_2}{L'_1 + L'_2} \right) \quad \ldots (5)$$

Apparatus

Optical bench; sphero-cylindrical lenses of positive focal power; circular apertures of varying diameter 2y; pinhole aperture; condenser lens.

Procedure

Use the condenser to focus light from the source on to the pinhole aperture so that this becomes the luminous object B. Place the sphero-cylindrical lens so that it forms line images at convenient distances l'_1 and l'_2 when B is at distance l from the sphero-cylindrical lens. With the use of a screen, observe how the cross section of the astigmatic beam changes along its axis and note the position l'_c of the disc of least confusion.

Measure the size of the two line foci and the diameter of the circle of least confusion. Place apertures of different diameter 2y in contact with the sphero-cylindrical lens and repeat these measurements. It may be easier to determine the size of the line foci if they are formed on graph paper screens.

Record your results as follows, taking four readings, and repeat for different object distances l.

1	2	3	4	5
Lens No.	Position of object	Position of sph.-cyl. lens	Position of first line focus	Position of second line focus

The difference between columns 3 and 2 gives l, between 4 and 3 l'_1, and between 5 and 3 l'_2. Hence from equations (1), (2) and (5) the size of the line foci and the circle of least confusion can be calculated and checked against the measured values. By application of conjugate foci for each principal meridian, the power of the sphero-cylindrical lens can be determined. Obtain the focal power of the lens by the use of a focimeter or by neutralization if you are not given its value.

EXPERIMENT 71B – THE TILTED SPHERICAL LENS

Theory

When light from a point source is incident normally on a spherical lens, the refracted beam is stigmatic, that is, it is brought to a point focus. If the lens is now tilted, the beam becomes astigmatic and exhibits the characteristics described previously.

It can be shown that a spherical lens of power F, if tilted through an angle θ, has a new spherical component

$$F_s = F \left(1 + \frac{\sin^2 \theta}{2n}\right)$$

where n is the refractive index of the lens, and a cylindrical component

$$F_c = F_s \tan^2 \theta$$

the axis being parallel to the axis of rotation.

Hence a + 6.00 sph. tilted 20 degrees about a horizontal axis has an effective power of nearly + 6.25/ + 0.75 × 180.

Procedure

Using the same apparatus and method as in Experiment 71a, determine the effective sphero-cylindrical power of a spherical lens of positive focal power tilted through angles of 10, 20 and 30 degrees. Compare your experimental determinations with the theoretical values obtained by calculation.

Experiment 72
THE DESIGN AND FORM OF SPHERICAL
OPHTHALMIC LENSES

Theory

It has been seen that in order for a spectacle lens to correct an eye, the back vertex focus of the lens must coincide with the eye's far point. The far point of an ametropic eye lies behind the eye in hypermetropia and in front in myopia. When the eye rotates behind a spectacle lens to view distant objects which are displaced from the eye's primary line, the far point also rotates, remaining at a fixed distance from the eye. We can imagine that as the far point rotates it traces out a spherical surface concentric with the eye's centre of rotation. This spherical surface is called the far point sphere (*Figure 72.1*).

The criterion for a best-form spectacle lens, used for distance vision, is that it should produce point images of distant point objects on the eye's far point sphere. The eye may be viewing along the optical axis of the lens or may rotate to view along an oblique direction, but in all cases the refracted pencil should be made to pass through the eye's centre of rotation and produce a point-focus on the far point sphere. It is convenient to assume the existence of a small aperture stop at the eye's centre of rotation since the complication of the rotating entrance pupil of the eye can then be ignored.

It was shown in Experiment 71b that when light passes obliquely through a spherical spectacle lens, the refracted pencil will be astigmatic. The great majority of best-form lenses are designed so that this defect of oblique astigmatism is zero, or has a minimum value, for a given stop position (the eye's centre of rotation is usually taken to be 27 mm behind the lens) and an angle of rotation of the eye in the region of 35 degrees. Unfortunately, with this point-focal type of spectacle lens, although the lens is designed to produce point images, these do not fall on but lie behind the eye's far point sphere. The discrepancy increases as the eye rotates further from the optical axis of the lens. The residual image shell error is normally ignored (*Figure 72.2*).

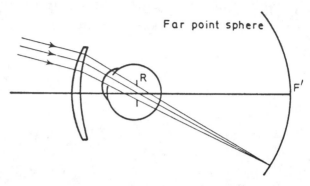

Figure 72.1. Diagram illustrating the criterion for a best-form spectacle lens. Narrow pencils of light, which may be incident axially or oblique, should be refracted to pass through the stop R, which is presumed to coincide with the eye's centre of rotation, and produce point images of distant point objects on the far point sphere

A second type of best-form lens is occasionally used in practice, the principle of which was first explained by Dr. Percival, an English ophthalmologist. If the bending of the point-focal lens is reduced somewhat, the tangential and sagittal line foci separate, the tangential focus lying closer to the lens (*Figure 72.3*). The lens now exhibits a small amount of astigmatism. If the bending is reduced — i.e., the lens is made flatter — by just the right amount to cause the tangential and sagittal foci to fall one on either side of the far point sphere and equidistant from it, the far point sphere will receive the disc of least confusion of the astigmatic pencil. If the astigmatism is small, the disc of least confusion will be small and may be perceived as a point. Lenses of this type are known as Percival lenses.

In the following experiment the tangential and sagittal powers are listed for various lens forms. These are measured from the vertex sphere, which is a spherical surface concentric with the eye's centre of rotation and having a radius equal to the distance from the centre of rotation to the back vertex of the lens. You should construct the image shell diagrams from these values in order to examine the performance of the lens. The radius of the vertex sphere may be taken as 27 mm.

Figure 72.2. Diagram illustrating the principle of the point-focal lens. The lens is designed to produce point images of distant point objects. These images, however, do not fall on the far point sphere. The surface marked P represents the shell upon which the point images may be considered to fall. The discrepancy between the two surfaces is referred to as image shell error

Figure 72.3. Diagram illustrating the principle of the Percival lens. The lens is designed to exhibit a small amount of oblique astigmatism such that the discs of least confusion of the astigmatic pencil fall on the far point sphere. The surfaces T and S represent the shells upon which the tangential and sagittal images may be considered to fall

Apparatus

Drawing instruments, reciprocal tables.

Procedure

(1)   Draw cross-sectional views of the lenses detailed below and construct to scale the optical axis, the vertex sphere, the position of the eye's centre of rotation and the far point sphere as shown in *Figure 72.4*.

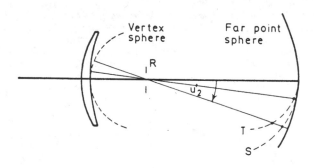

Figure 72.4

(2)   Obtain the reciprocals of the tangential and sagittal powers, F'_T and F'_S respectively, in order to obtain the tangential and sagittal oblique vertex sphere focal lengths (f'_T and f'_S).

(3)   Measuring from the vertex sphere through the centre of rotation, locate the positions of the tangential and sagittal foci for each angle of rotation, u'_2.

(4)   Draw a smooth curve joining the tangential foci to obtain the tangential image shell T.

(5)   Draw a smooth curve joining the sagittal foci to obtain the sagittal image shell S.

(6)   Discuss the optical performance of each lens form and explain how each form departs from the criterion for a best-form lens.

Lens data

(1) Back vertex power   + 5.00 D
     Back surface power   − 2.00 D
     Front surface power   + 6.84 D
     Axial thickness   5 mm

u'_2	F'_T	F'_S
5°	+ 5.02	+ 5.00
10°	+ 5.07	+ 5.00
15°	+ 5.16	+ 5.01
20°	+ 5.29	+ 5.01
25°	+ 5.46	+ 5.01
30°	+ 5.66	+ 5.01
35°	+ 5.91	+ 5.00

(2) Back vertex power   + 5.00 D
     Back surface power   − 4.00 D
     Front surface power   + 8.74 D
     Axial thickness   5 mm

u'_2	F'_T	F'_S
5°	+ 5.01	+ 5.00
10°	+ 5.02	+ 4.99
15°	+ 5.05	+ 4.97
20°	+ 5.08	+ 4.94
25°	+ 5.11	+ 4.91
30°	+ 5.13	+ 4.86
35°	+ 5.15	+ 4.79

(3) Back vertex power   + 5.00 D
     Back surface power   − 6.00 D
     Front surface power   + 10.62 D
     Axial thickness   5 mm

u'_2	F'_T	F'_S
5°	+ 5.00	+ 4.99
10°	+ 4.98	+ 4.97
15°	+ 4.96	+ 4.94
20°	+ 4.92	+ 4.89
25°	+ 4.87	+ 4.83
30°	+ 4.79	+ 4.75
35°	+ 4.68	+ 4.65

(4) Back vertex power   − 4.00 D
     Back surface power   − 6.00 D
     Front surface power   + 2.00 D
     Axial thickness   1.2 mm

u'_2	F'_T	F'_S
5°	− 4.01	− 4.00
10°	− 4.05	− 4.00
15°	− 4.11	− 4.01
20°	− 4.18	− 4.01
25°	− 4.28	− 4.01
30°	− 4.38	− 4.01
35°	− 4.47	− 3.99

Experiment 73
BLANK SELECTION.
NOMINAL SURFACE POWERS

Theory

Blank. A piece of glass or plastics material for the making of a lens at any stage before completion of the surfacing processes.

Semi-finished blank. A blank having one side completely surfaced.

Semi-finished sphere. A semi-finished blank whose convex surface has been completely worked spherical.

Semi-finished toric. A semi-finished blank where one surface has been completely worked toroidal.

The great majority of single-vision lenses which pass through the surfacing workshop are semi-finished blanks, where the first side has been completed by the blank manufacturer and the final prescription is to be obtained by completing the second side.

The object of this exercise is to determine the base curve which must be used for a given prescription and to write out the nominal surface powers using this base.

Table 73.1 indicates the base curve which should be used for prescriptions in the range − 12.00 D sph. to + 6.00 D sph., astigmatic prescription being considered in minus-cylinder transposition.

In cases where two lenses in a given prescription require different base curves owing to differing powers it is usual to match the base curves by choosing the more convex curve for each lens.

The prescriptions given below must be written out with the convex surface above the line and the concave surface below the line, using the normal rules for thin lens transposition.

TABLE 73.1. BLANK SELECTION

Nominal base	To work powers
+ 2.00	− 9.25 to − 12.00
+ 3.00	− 6.25 to − 9.00
+ 4.00	− 2.25 to − 6.00
+ 6.00	− 2.00 to + 1.00
+ 7.00	+ 1.25 to + 3.00
+ 8.00	+ 3.25 to + 4.00
+ 9.00	+ 4.25 to + 5.00
+ 10.00	+ 5.25 to + 6.00

Procedure

(1) Transpose the astigmatic prescriptions, if necessary, to minus-cylinder form.

(2) Use the sphere of the minus-cylinder prescription in conjunction with *Table 73.1* to determine the nominal base curves which are to be used. Check both right and left lenses to ensure that the base curves match. If not, use the rule given above.

(3) Using the minus-cylinder transposition write out the nominal surface powers, assuming that semi-finished sphere blanks are to be used.

(4) Transpose any astigmatic prescriptions to plus-cylinder form and write out the nominal surface powers, assuming that semi-finished toric blanks (with plus base curves) are to be used.

Note. − Omit step 4 for spherical prescriptions.

Examples

(1) R. + 2.00   L. + 3.00/− 0.50 X 180

Nominal bases: R. + 7.00   L. + 7.00

Semi-finished meniscus

R. $\dfrac{+ 7.00}{- 5.00}$ L. $\dfrac{+ 7.00}{- 4.00 \times 90 / - 4.50 \times 180}$

Semi-finished toric

R. $\dfrac{+ 7.00}{- 5.00}$ L. $\dfrac{+ 7.00 \times 180 / + 7.50 \times 90}{- 4.50}$

(2)   R. $-2.00/+1.00 \times 45$ L. $-2.75/+0.25 \times 135$

Nominal bases: R. $+6.00$ L. $+6.00$

Semi-finished meniscus

R. $\dfrac{+6.00}{-7.00 \times 45/-8.00 \times 135}$ L. $\dfrac{+6.00}{-8.50 \times 135/-8.75 \times 45}$

Semi-finished toric

R. $\dfrac{+6.00 \times 135/+7.00 \times 45}{-8.00}$ L. $\dfrac{+6.00 \times 45/+6.25 \times 135}{-8.75}$

Prescriptions

(1)   R. $+4.00/+1.00 \times 90$ L. $+3.50$
(2)   R. $-1.00/-1.00 \times 180$ L. $-1.50/-0.75 \times 180$
(3)   R. $+4.50/+0.50 \times 30$ L. $+5.25/+0.25 \times 150$
(4)   R. $-9.50/-0.50 \times 45$ L. $-8.00/-0.75 \times 135$
(5)   R. $+0.25/+0.25 \times 15$ L. $-0.75/+0.25 \times 180$
(6)   R. -1.75 L. $-1.75/-1.25 \times 70$

Experiment 74
THICKNESS OF MINUS LENSES

Theory

The centre thickness of a minus lens can be determined from $t = 2 + 0.2$ F, where F is the spherical power of the lens in minus-cylinder transposition. The minimum permissible centre thickness is 1.0 mm and this would be applied to all lenses over -5.00 D.

Table 74.1 can be used to determine the centre thickness of minus lenses. The thickness of a lens is normally specified to the nearest 0.1 mm and it is conventional to round 0.25 powers up to the nearest 0.1 mm, e.g. -0.25, 2.0 mm; -0.75, 1.9 mm; etc.

TABLE 74.1

Sph. power	Sph. or cyl. lenses
-0.50	1.9
-1.00	1.8
-1.50	1.7
-2.00	1.6
-2.50	1.5
-3.00	1.4
-3.50	1.3
-4.00	1.2
-4.50	1.1
-5.00	1.0
over -5.00	1.0

The relationship between the edge and centre thickness of minus lenses can be deduced from the geometry of *Figure 74.1*, where it can be seen that the edge thickness equals the sag of the concave surface minus the sag of the convex surface plus the centre thickness, i.e.

$$e = s_2 - s_1 + t$$

Figure 74.1

The purpose of this exercise is to determine the edge thickness of various minus lenses, assuming that astigmatic lenses will be made as plus or minus base torics. The forms of the lenses can be obtained from the following blank selection chart (*Table 74.2*), remembering that it is applied to the sphere in minus-cylinder transposition.

TABLE 74.2

Nominal base	To work powers
+ 2.00	− 9.25 to − 12.00
+ 3.00	− 6.25 to − 9.00
+ 4.00	− 2.25 to − 6.00
+ 6.00	− 0.25 to − 2.00

The sag of each surface is to be read from sag tables.* Assume that spectacle crown glass (n = 1.523) is used.

Procedure

(1)   Transpose the prescription, if necessary, to the minus-cylinder form and use the sphere to determine the nominal base curve.

(2)   Use the sphere (i.e. spherical power) of the minus-cylinder transposition to determine the centre thickness of the lens, t.

(3)   Write out the nominal surface powers of the lens assuming that a semi-finished sphere blank is to be used.

Tables for Surfacing Instruction, M. Jalie, IPC Business Press, 1972.

(4) Find the sag s_1 of the convex surface at the specified diameter, using the sag tables.

(5) Find the sag s_2 of the concave surface from the sag tables. If the lens is astigmatic find the sags of both the concave base curve and cross curve.

(6) Find the edge thickness from $e = s_2 - s_1 + t$. If the lens is astigmatic there will be two values for e:

$$e_{thin} = s_{2\ base} - s_1 + t$$

$$e_{thick} = s_{2\ cross} s_1 + t$$

rounding the final answers to the nearest 0.1 mm.

(7) Write out the nominal surface powers assuming that a semi-finished toric blank is to be used for the astigmatic prescriptions. Note that the base curve and sphere curve sags will be the same as the sags found for the sphere curve and cross curve in (4) and (5) above, and, therefore, c_{thick} will be the same for each form.

(8) Find the sag of the convex cross curve from the sag table.

For plus base toric minus lenses:

$$e_{thin} = s_2 \quad s_{1\ cross} + t$$

$$e_{thick} = s_2 - s_{1\ base} + t$$

Work through the two examples below to confirm the procedure.

Examples

(1) Rx. $- 3.00$ Blank diameter: 60 mm

Nominal base: $+ 4.00$ Form: $\dfrac{+ 4.00}{- 7.00}$

Centre thickness: 1.4 mm

Sag 4.00 at 60 = 3.49 mm

Sag 7.00 at 60 = 6.29 mm

$e = 6.29 - 3.49 + 1.4 = 4.2$ mm

(2) Rx. $- 4.00/- 2.50 \times 180$ 56 mm round blank

Nominal base: $+ 4.00$

Centre thickness: 1.2 mm

255

Semi-finished meniscus form

$$\frac{+4.00}{-8.00 \times 90/-10.50 \times 180}$$

Sag 4.00 at 56 = 3.03 mm

Sag 8.00 at 56 = 6.30 mm

Sag 10.50 at 56 = 8.62 mm

e_{thin} = 6.30 − 3.03 + 1.2 = 4.5 mm

e_{thick} = 8.62 − 3.03 + 1.2 = 6.8 mm

Semi-finished toric form

$$\frac{+4.00 \times 180/+6.50 \times 90}{-10.50}$$

Sag 6.50 at 56 = 5.03 mm

e_{thin} = 8.62 − 5.03 + 1.2 = 4.8 mm

e_{thick} = 8.62 − 3.03 + 1.2 = 6.8 mm

Prescriptions

(1)	− 2.00 DS	60 mm round blank
(2)	− 7.00/+ 1.00 × 90	52 mm round blank
(3)	− 3.25/+ 0.75 × 45	58 mm round blank
(4)	− 5.00/− 1.50 × 90	56 × 50 mm rectangular blank
(5)	− 0.25/− 0.50 × 30	60 mm round blank

Experiment 75
THICKNESS OF PLUS UNCUT LENSES

Theory

The optimum value for the thickness of a plus lens depends eventually upon the diameter of the edged lens and the type of glazing. In this exercise it is assumed that the details of the frame are unknown and that we are concerned only with uncut lenses.

The edge thickness of a plus uncut lens can be determined from *Table 75.1*, in which the plus power given refers for astigmatic lenses to the sphere in the minus-cylinder transposition. 0.25 D intervals should be rounded up to the nearest 0.1 mm, e.g. + 0.25, 2.0 mm; + 0.75, 1.9 mm, etc.

TABLE 75.1

Sph. power	Edge thickness
Plano	2.0
+ 0.50	1.9
+ 1.00	1.8
+ 1.50	1.7
+ 2.00	1.6
+ 2.50	1.5
+ 3.00	1.4
+ 3.50	1.3
+ 4.00	1.2
+ 4.50	1.1
+ 5.00 to + 9.75	1.0
+ 10.00 and over	0.5

The relationship between the centre thickness and the edge thickness of a plus lens can be seen, from the geometry of *Figure 75.1*, to be: centre thickness equals the sag of the convex curve minus the sag of the concave curve plus the edge thickness, i.e.

$$t = s_1 - s_2 + e$$

Figure 75.1

The purpose of this exercise is to determine the centre thickness of various plus uncut lenses assuming that astigmatic lenses will be made as plus or minus base torics and that the nominal surface powers are actually worked. Also the thick edge substance is to be found.

The forms of the lenses can be obtained from the following blank selection chart (*Table 75.2*), remembering that it applies to the sphere of an astigmatic prescription in minus-cylinder transposition.

TABLE 75.2

Nominal base	To work powers
+ 6.00	Plano to + 1.00
+ 7.00	+ 1.25 to + 3.00
+ 8.00	+ 3.25 to + 4.00
+ 9.00	+ 4.25 to + 5.00
+ 10.00	+ 5.25 to + 6.00

The sag of each surface is to be read from sag tables. Assume that spectacle crown glass, n = 1.523, is used.

Procedure

(1) Transpose the prescription, if necessary, to the minus- cylinder form and use the sphere to determine the nominal base curve.

(2) Use the sphere of the minus-cylinder prescription to determine the edge thickness of the lens.

(3)   Write out the nominal surface powers of the lens assuming that a rough meniscus blank is to be used.

(4)   Find the sag s_1 of the convex surface at the specified diameter, using the sag tables.

(5)   Find the sag s_2 of the concave surface from the sag tables. If the lens is astigmatic find the sags of both the concave base curve and cross curve.

(6)   Find the centre thickness from $t = s_1 - s_2 + e$. If the lens is astigmatic, s_2 must be the sag of the base curve. Round the centre thickness to the nearest 0.1 mm.

(7)   In the case of astigmatic lenses, find the thick edge substances from $e_{thick} = t - (s_1 - s_2{}_{cross})$.

(8)   Transpose the prescription, if necessary, to the plus-cylinder form and write out the nominal surface powers assuming that a semi-finished toric blank is to be used for the astigmatic prescriptions. Note that the base curve and the sphere curve sags will be the same as the sags found for the sphere curve and the cross curve in 4 and 5 above, providing, of course, that the blank is circular.

(9)   Find the sag of the convex cross curve from the sag tables.

For plus base torics:

$$t = s_1{}_{cross} - s_2 + e$$

$$e_{thick} = t - (s_1{}_{base} - s_2)$$

Work through the example below to confirm the procedure.

Example

Rx. + 4.00/+ 1.00 × 90   Blank diameter: 60 mm

Nominal base: + 9.00

Edge thickness: 1.0 mm

Semi-finished meniscus form $\dfrac{+ 9.00}{- 4.00 \times 90/ - 5.00 \times 180}$

Sag 9.00 at 60 = 8.34 mm

Sag 4.00 at 60 = 3.49 mm

Sag 5.00 at 60 = 4.39 mm

t = 8.34 − 3.49 + 1.0 = 5.9 mm

e_{thick} = 5.9 − (8.34 − 4.39) = 1.9 mm

Semi-finished toric form

$$\frac{+9.00 \times 180/+10.00 \times 90}{-5.00}$$

Sag 10.00 at 60 = 9.46 mm

$t = 9.46 - 4.39 + 1.0 = 6.1$ mm

$e_{thick} = 6.1 - (8.34 - 4.39) = 2.1$ mm

Prescriptions

(1)	+ 2.00 DS	58 mm round blank
(2)	+ 3.50/+ 1.50 × 90	60 mm round blank
(3)	+ 0.25/+ 0.50 × 45	56 mm round blank
(4)	+ 1.75/+ 0.75 × 60	50 mm round blank
(5)	Plano/+ 4.00 × 180	56 × 52 mm rectangular blank

Experiment 76
PLUS LENSES: FRONT SURFACE
COMPENSATION

Theory

Nominal or uncompensated surface power. The hypothetical surface power which would be worked if the lens thickness is ignored.

Compensated or reduced surface power. The actual surface power which must be worked taking the effect of the lens thickness into account.

Vertex power allowance (VPA). The difference between the compensated and nominal curves.

The back vertex power of a lens depends not only upon the lens surface powers but also upon its centre thickness. In minus lenses without prism the effect of the lens thickness is negligible and nominal transposition is sufficient to determine the surface powers. When the centre thickness exceeds 2 mm, however, it is necessary to compensate one of the surfaces to allow for the effect of the thickness. The amount of compensation which has to be added to the nominal or uncompensated surface power to produce the compensated or reduced surface power is called the *vertex power allowance* (VPA). The VPA is always negative, that is the reduced front curve is always less positive, or the reduced back curve is always more negative, than the nominal curve. In determining the compensated surface power it is necessary to bear in mind the tolerances which are allowed in the lens power (B.S. 2738, *Spectacle Lenses*) and the available tool range. For the purposes of this exercise it will be assumed that tools are available in 0.12 D intervals. The type of blank which is considered in this exercise is a semi-finished minus base toric where the manufacturer has completed the back surface with a − 3.00 base curve and a range of cross curves from − 3.25 DC to

− 9.25 DC. We can, therefore, produce cylinders up to − 6.00 DC. We will also assume that a − 3.00 spherical curve is available.

The following procedure is designed to produce uncut lenses up to + 8.00 sphere with any minus cylinder.

No blank selection table is required since all lenses are made on a − 3.00 base. The thin-edge substance can be assumed to be 1.0 mm in each case. The centre thickness of the lens, the compensated front curve and the thick-edge substance are to be determined.

Procedure

(1) Transpose the prescription, if necessary, to the minus-cylinder transposition.

(2) Find the sag of the sphere at the specified diameter using the sag tables.

(3) Add 1.0 mm to the sag of the sphere and round the result UPWARDS to the nearest 0.5 mm.

(4) Write out the nominal surface powers of the lens using a − 3.00 D base curve.

(5) Using the vertex power allowance table find the VPA for the nominal front surface power and the rounded centre thickness. (Remember that this quantity is normally negative but it is unlikely that the minus sign is printed in the tables.)

(6) Compensate the front surface by subtracting the VPA (ignoring signs) from the nominal front curve and round the result to the nearest 0.12 interval.

(7) Write out the true surface powers of the lens.

(8) Find the sag s_1 of the convex surface at the specified diameter from the sag tables (it will be necessary to estimate 0.12 D curves).

(9) Find the sag s_2 of the 3.00 D base curve at the specified diameter. If the lens is astigmatic find the sag of the concave cross curve.

(10) Find the thin edge substance from $e_{thin} = t - (s_1 - s_{2\ base})$. If the lens is astigmatic find the thick edge substance from $e_{thick} = t - (s_1 - s_{2\ cross})$; round each value to the nearest 0.1 mm.

Work through the example below to confirm the procedure.

Example

+ 5.00/− 1.00 × 90   Blank diameter: 60 mm

Sag 5.00 at 60 = 4.39 mm

t = 4.39 + 1.0 = 5.39 mm (round to 5.5 mm)

Nominal surface powers: $\dfrac{+\,8.00}{-\,3.00 \times 180/-\,4.00 \times 90}$

VPA (nominal + 8.00, t = 5.5) = 0.22 (round to 0.25)

Actual surface powers: $\dfrac{+\,7.75}{-\,3.00 \times 180/-\,4.00 \times 90}$

Sag 7.75 at 60 = 7.03 mm

Sag 3.00 at 60 = 2.60 mm

Sag 4.00 at 60 = 3.49 mm

e_{thin} = 5.5 − (7.03 − 2.60) = 1.1 mm

e_{thick} = 5.5 − (7.03 − 3.49) = 2.0 mm

Prescriptions

(1)	+ 6.00/− 2.00 × 90	60 mm round blank
(2)	+ 6.50/+ 1.50 × 45	56 mm round blank
(3)	+ 5.50	52 mm round blank
(4)	+ 4.75/+ 1.25 × 30	58 mm round blank
(5)	+ 2.25/+ 4.50 × 180	56 × 52 mm rectangular blank

Experiment 77
PLUS LENSES: BACK SURFACE POWER,
SEMI-FINISHED SPHERES

Theory

In order to reduce the number of tools which the surfacing workshop
must carry, some blank manufacturers supply semi-finished blanks
where the convex surface already incorporates an arbitrary compensation. Thus a packet marked with a + 10.00 D nominal base curve
might contain a blank whose base curve is actually + 9.62, the manufacturer having added a vertex power allowance of − 0.38 D to the
convex surface. Although the vertex power allowance can be exactly
correct for only one particular centre thickness, small variations in the
centre thickness from the exact value will produce only small errors in
back vertex power. Providing that these errors do not exceed the
permissible tolerances this system offers a convenient method for
surfacing plus lenses.

Table 77.1 shows the nominal base, actual base, exact centre thickness and the safe range of centre thicknesses for the stated error for a
typical series of semi-finished sphere blanks.

TABLE 77.1

Nominal base	Actual base	Centre thickness, mm		Error	To work powers
		Exact	*Range*		
+ 6.00	+ 5.94	2.6	0 − 5.1	± 0.06	Plano to + 1.00
+ 7.00	+ 6.90	3.2	1.3 − 5.0	± 0.06	+ 1.25 to + 3.00
+ 8.00	+ 7.80	4.9	3.5 − 6.3	± 0.06	+ 3.25 to + 4.00
+ 9.00	+ 8.75	4.8	2.6 − 7.0	± 0.12	+ 4.25 to + 5.00
+ 10.00	+ 9.62	6.0	4.2 − 7.8	± 0.12	+ 5.25 to + 6.00
+ 11.50	+ 10.80	8.6	7.2 − 9.9	± 0.12	+ 6.25 to + 8.00

The purpose of this exercise is to use *Table 77.1* in conjunction with the table of sags, to determine the surface powers, centre and edge thicknesses of plus uncut lenses up to 8.00 D with any minus cylinder.

For astigmatic prescriptions the cylinder will be incorporated as a minus base toric on the back surface. The procedure outlined below should enable the thin edge substance to lie within 0.1 mm of the value stipulated in step 3.

Procedure

(1)   Transpose the prescription, if necessary, to the minus-cylinder transposition.

(2)   Find the sag of the sphere at the specified diameter using the sag tables, and round to the nearest 0.1 mm.

(3)   Use *Table 77.2* to determine the thin-edge substance from the sphere of the minus-cylinder transposition rounding 0.25 intervals up to the nearest 0.1 mm. Add to the sag found in step 2 to obtain the centre thickness t.

TABLE 77.2

Sphere power	Edge thickness
Plano	2.0
+ 0.50	1.9
+ 1.00	1.8
+ 1.50	1.7
+ 2.00	1.6
+ 2.50	1.5
+ 3.00	1.4
+ 3.50	1.3
+ 4.00	1.2
+ 4.50	1.1
+ 5.00 to + 8.00	1.0

(4)   Check, using *Table 77.1*, that the centre thickness lies within the safe range for the sphere power required. IF NOT, DO NOT PROCEED. (The blank is unsuitable for this method of working and further compensation is required on the concave surface; see Experiment 83.)

(5)   Write out the surface powers for the lens, assuming that a semi-finished sphere blank is to be used, but substituting the actual convex surface power given in *Table 77.1* instead of the nominal front surface power. These are the actual surface powers required.

(6)   Find the sag s_1 of the convex surface at the specified diameter from the sag tables. It will be necessary to estimate most sags by comparing adjacent values.

(7)   Find the sag s_2 of the concave base curve at the specified diameter. If the lens is astigmatic find the sag of the concave cross curve.

(8)   Find the thin edge substance from $e_{thin} = t - (s_1 - s_{2\ base})$. If the lens is astigmatic find the thick edge substance from $e_{thick} = t - (s_1 - s_{2\ cross})$. If e_{thin} differs by more than 0.1 mm from the required value add the difference to the edge and centre substances to correct this and again check that the centre thickness is within the safe range from *Table 77.1*. Work through the following example to confirm the procedure.

Example

+ 3.50/+ 1.50 × 90 .   56 mm round blank

Minus-cylinder transposition = + 5.00/− 1.50 × 180

Sag 5.00 at 56 = 3.8 mm

t = 3.8 + 1 = 4.8 mm

Actual surface powers: $\dfrac{+\ 8.75}{-\ 4.00 \times 90/-\ 5.50 \times 180}$

Sag 8.75 at 56 = 6.96 mm

Sag 4.00 at 56 = 3.03 mm

Sag 5.50 at 56 = 4.22 mm

e_{thin} = 4.8 − (6.96 − 3.03) = 0.9 mm

e_{thick} = 4.8 − (6.96 − 4.22) = 2.1 mm

Prescriptions

(1)	+ 3.00	60 mm round blank
(2)	+ 5.50/+ 2.50 × 90	56 mm round blank
(3)	+ 0.25/+ 0.25 × 45	58 mm round blank
(4)	− 2.00/+ 4.00 × 60	70 mm round blank
(5)	+ 1.50/+ 0.75 × 90	56 × 52 mm rectangular blank

Experiment 78
PLUS LENSES: BACK SURFACE POWER, SEMI-FINISHED TORICS

Theory

The semi-finished toric blank considered in this exercise is a semi-finished blank whose convex surface has been completely finished as a plus base toric. It is designed only for producing astigmatic lenses. Compensation is provided by the manufacturer on both the base curve and the cross curve. Since these curves differ, the compensation for the base curve differs from the compensation for the cross curve. It is necessary to know both these curves in order to be able to control the thin edge substance.

Table 78.1 shows the nominal base, actual base, exact centre thickness and the safe range of centre thicknesses for the stated error for a typical series of semi-finished toric blanks. The actual cross curve depends upon the cylinder power and this must be determined when the blank is selected either from the information on the packet or by means of a sagometer.

TABLE 78.1

Nominal base	Actual base	Centre thickness, mm		Error	To work powers
		Exact	Range		
+ 6.00	+ 5.94	2.6	0 – 5.1	± 0.06	Plano to + 1.50
+ 7.50	+ 7.37	3.6	2.0 – 5.1	± 0.06	+ 1.75 to + 3.75
+ 9.00	+ 8.75	4.8	2.6 – 7.0	± 0.12	+ 4.00 to + 5.00
+ 10.25	+ 9.87	5.7	4.0 – 7.4	± 0.12	+ 5.25 to + 6.00
+ 11.50	+ 10.80	8.6	7.2 – 9.9	± 0.12	+ 6.25 to + 8.00

267

When selecting blanks from this table it should be noted that the sphere must be taken from the plus-cylinder transposition of the prescription. The purpose of this exercise is to determine, with the aid of a table of sags, the surface powers, centre and edge thicknesses of plus uncut lenses up to + 8.00 D with any plus cylinder. The thin edge will normally be found to lie within 0.1 mm of the value stipulated in step 3.

Procedure

(1) Transpose the prescription, if necessary, to the minus-cylinder transposition.

(2) Find the sag of the sphere at the specified diameter using the sag tables and round to the nearest 0.1 mm.

(3) Use *Table 78.2* to determine the thin edge substance from the sphere of the minus-cylinder transposition, rounding 0.25 intervals up to the nearest 0.1 mm. Add to the sag found in step 2 to obtain the centre thickness t.

TABLE 78.2

Sphere power	Edge thickness
Plano	2.0
+ 0.50	1.9
+ 1.00	1.8
+ 1.50	1.7
+ 2.00	1.6
+ 2.50	1.5
+ 3.00	1.4
+ 3.50	1.3
+ 4.00	1.2
+ 4.50	1.1
+ 5.00 to + 8.00	1.0

(4) Transpose the prescription to the plus-cylinder form.

(5) Check that the centre thickness lies within the safe range for the sphere power required (from the plus-cylinder form of the prescription). IF NOT, DO NOT PROCEED (the blank is unsuitable for this method of working, further compensation being required on the concave surface).

(6) Write out the surface powers for the lens assuming that a semi-finished toric blank is to be used but substituting the actual base curve and actual cross curve given with each prescription.

The sphere curve obtained is the actual back curve which must be worked.

(7)   Find the sags of the base curve and the cross curve from the table of sags, $s_{1\ base}$ and $s_{1\ cross}$. It will be necessary to estimate most of these by comparing adjacent values.

(8)   Find the sag s_2 of the concave sphere curve.

(9)   Find the thin edge substance from $e_{thin} = t - (s_{1\ cross} - s_2)$ and the thick edge substance from $e_{thick} = t - (s_{1\ base} - s_2)$. If e_{thin} differs by more than 0.1 mm from the required value adjust e_{thin}, e_{thick} and t to correct this and again check that the centre thickness lies within the safe range from *Table 78.1*.

Work through the following example to confirm the procedure.

Example

+ 4.50/+ 1.00 × 90   52 mm round blank

Blank curves: + 8.75/+ 9.69

Minus-cylinder transposition = + 5.50/− 1.00 × 180

Sag 5.50 at 52 = 3.6 mm

t = 3.6 + 1 = 4.6 mm

Plus-cylinder transposition = + 4.50/+ 1.00 × 90

Actual surface powers: $\dfrac{+\ 8.75 \times 180/+\ 9.69 \times 90}{-\ 4.50}$

Sag 8.75 at 52 = 5.95 mm

Sag 9.69 at 52 = 6.6 mm (estimated)

Sag 4.50 at 52 = 2.95 mm

e_{thin} = 4.6 − (6.6 − 2.95) = 1.0 mm

e_{thick} = 4.6 − (5.95 − 2.95) = 1.6 mm

Prescriptions

(1)   + 0.50/+ 0.50 × 90   60 mm round blank
       Blank curves + 5.94/+ 6.43

(2)   + 2.50/+ 1.50 × 45   58 mm round blank
       Blank curves + 7.37/+ 8.81

(3)   + 5.25/+ 3.00 × 180   52 mm round blank
       Blank curves + 9.87/+ 12.62

269

(4)   + 4.50/− 0.75 × 30   56 mm round blank
      Blank curves + 7.37/+ 8.09
(5)   + 10.50/− 4.00 × 120   52 mm round blank
      Blank curves + 10.80/+ 14.25

Experiment 79
SPHERICAL PRISMATIC LENSES.
SEMI-FINISHED SPHERES

Theory

When a prescription includes prismatic effect which cannot be obtained by decentration it is necessary to incorporate the prism by working the refracting surfaces at an angle to one another. The prism is controlled by ensuring that one edge of the blank remains thicker than the opposite edge, along the base-apex direction, by an amount known as the thickness difference g. The necessary thickness difference for various powers of prism at different diameters is provided in the surfacing tables. Sometimes two prismatic components are required for a given lens, one vertical and one horizontal. In these cases the two components must be compounded into a single prismatic effect before proceeding.

The purpose of this exercise is to obtain complete surfacing data for spherical lenses which include worked prism, assuming that semi-finished sphere blanks are to be used. In addition to finding the surface powers and centre thickness for each lens the prism thickness difference must be determined along the base-apex direction and the edge thickness at $90°$ to the base-apex direction, thus providing four calipering points on the edge of the uncut. In plus uncut lenses the centre thickness must be increased by half the thickness difference of the prism at the uncut diameter. It is necessary to check the centre thickness range in order to ensure that the power remains within the recommended tolerance.

In minus lenses the increase in thickness at the geometrical centre should be determined by adding the *smaller* of the two quantities (a) and (b):

271

(a)   Half the thickness difference of the prism at the uncut diameter.

(b) $- P^2/10F$, where P is the prism power and F is the spherical power (or 'sphere') of the prescription.

The necessary information relating to blank selection, actual base
The necessary information relating to blank selection, actual base
curves and minimum centre or edge thicknesses is given in Experiment 74 for minus lenses and Experiment 77 for plus lenses.

You may assume that the base curves + 2.00, + 3.00 and + 4.00 (for negative prescriptions) are the true curves on the blanks.

Procedure

(1)   If both vertical and horizontal prisms have been prescribed, compound these into a single resultant prism, rounding the resultant to the nearest $0.12^\triangle$ if up to $2^\triangle$ or to the nearest $0.25^\triangle$ if over $2^\triangle$.

(2)   Find the thickness difference, g, of the prism at the blank diameter from the thickness difference table.

(3)   If the sphere is negative, compute the quantity $- P^2/10F$. Compare this value with half the thickness difference obtained in step 2. The smaller of these two quantities must be added to the centre thickness of the lens selected from *Table 74.1* to find the geometric centre thickness t.

(4)   If the sphere is positive find the edge thickness from Experiment 77; add half the prism thickness difference obtained in step 2, and the sag of the sphere at the blank diameter; read from the sag tables to obtain the centre thickness t.

(5)   Round the centre thickness to the nearest 0.1 mm and check, from the information given in Experiment 77, that it lies within the safe range for the sphere power required. IF NOT, DO NOT PROCEED.

(6)   Write out the surface powers for the lens, substituting the actual convex surface power given in *Table 77.1* instead of the nominal front surface power. These are the actual surface powers required.

(7)   Find the sag s_1 of the convex surface at the specified diameter, from the sag table.

(8)   Find the sag s_2 of the concave surface at the specified diameter.

(9)   If the sphere is negative find the edge thickness at $90°$ to the base-apex direction from $e = s_2 - s_1 + t$, where t is the geometric centre thickness found in step 3. To find the thick-edge substance along the base-apex direction add half the prism thickness difference found in step 2 to the value of e found above. To find the thin-edge substance along the base-apex direction subtract the thickness difference found in step 2 from the thick-edge substance.

272

This completes the procedure for a negative lens.

(10) If the sphere is positive find the thin edge substance along the base-apex direction from

$$e = t - g/2 - (s_1 - s_2)$$

where $g/2$ is half the prism thickness difference obtained in step 2. If this value of e differs by more than 0.1 mm from the required value add the difference to the edge and centre thicknesses to correct these and again ensure that the centre thickness lies within the safe range given in *Table 77.1*.

(11) Find the thick-edge substance along the base-apex direction by adding the thickness difference g to the thin-edge substance.

(12) Find the edge thickness at $90°$ to the base-apex direction by adding half the thickness difference to the thin-edge substance.

Work through the following examples to confirm the procedure.

Examples

(1) -4.00 ◯ $3^\triangle$ base IN   56 mm round blank

Thickness difference, $3^\triangle$ prism at 56 = 3.2 mm

Half this value is 1.6 mm

$-P^2/10F = 9/40 = 0.23$, which is smaller than 1.6, so that the centre thickness $t = 1.2 + 0.2 = 1.4$ mm.

Surface powers: $\dfrac{+4.00}{-8.00}$

Sag 4.00 at 56 = 3.0 mm

Sag 8.00 at 56 = 6.3 mm

At $90°$ to base-apex direction e $= 6.3 - 3.0 + 1.4 = 4.7$ mm

Along base-apex direction $e_{thick} = 4.7 + 1.6 = 6.3$ mm

$\qquad\qquad\qquad e_{thin} = 6.3 - 3.2 = 3.1$ mm

(2) $+5.00$ ◯ $1\frac{1}{2}^\triangle$ UP and $2^\triangle$ IN   58 mm round blank

Resultant prism = $2\frac{1}{2}^\triangle$ base 37

Thickness difference, $2\frac{1}{2}^\triangle$ prism at 58 = 2.8 mm

Half this value is 1.4 mm

Edge thickness = 1.0 mm

Sag 5.00 at 58 = 4.1 mm

273

$t = 1.0 + 1.4 + 4.1 = 6.5$ mm   (safe range $= 2.6 - 7.0$ mm)

Surface powers: $\dfrac{+8.75}{-4.00}$

Sag 8.75 at 58 $= 7.5$ mm

Sag 4.00 at 58 $= 3.3$ mm

$e_{thin} = 6.5 - 1.4 - (7.5 - 3.3) = 0.9$ mm

$e_{thick} = 0.9 + 2.8 = 3.7$ mm

At $90°$ to base-apex direction $e = 0.9 + 1.4 = 2.3$ mm

Prescriptions

(1)	-0.50 ◯	$4^\triangle$ base UP	60 mm round blank
(2)	-8.00 ◯	$5^\triangle$ base IN	52 mm round blank
(3)	$+1.00$ ◯	$2^\triangle$ UP & $3^\triangle$ IN	56 mm round blank
(4)	$+7.00$ ◯	$5^\triangle$ OUT	52 mm round blank
(5)	$+0.25$ ◯	$3^\triangle$ DOWN	60 mm round blank

Experiment 80
SHAPED PLUS LENSES.
SEMI-FINISHED SPHERES

Theory

When details of the finished lens shape and size are known it is possible to determine the minimum centre thickness for the lens which will produce the required edge thickness at a specified diameter. This problem usually arises when the lens includes a strong cylinder or prism. Prismatic lenses are dealt with in a future exercise.

The method described in this exercise is the '3-meridian' method, which enables us to determine fairly accurately which meridian controls the thickness of a shaped lens. When this meridian has been determined we can find the edge thickness along the minus axis meridian of the blank.

Notional Lens Power

Consider the prescription + 2.00/+ 4.00 X 90, whose principal powers are represented by the optical cross:

Figure 80.1
275

So far as the thickness of the lens is concerned we can consider that, since the power of the lens along 90 is + 2.00 and along 180 is + 6.00, along the 45 or 135 meridian midway between 90 and 180 the power of the lens will be + 4.00. This is made up from the power of the sphere + 2.00, and half the power of the cylinder since the meridian in question lies halfway between the 90 and 180 meridians of the lens. The notional power of a cylinder, F_θ, along a meridian inclined at an angle θ to the axis meridian of the cylinder whose power is denoted by F, can be found from

$$F_\theta = F\sin^2 \theta$$

Values of F_θ are normally available in surfacing tables.

Suppose now that the prescription + 2.00/4.00 × 90 is required for a 52 × 44 Quadra shape as shown in *Figure 80.2*. The distances from the standard optical centre position (SOCP) to the edges of the lens are shown along the two power meridians, 90 and 180, and along the longest meridian of the shape, which lies at 30° to the + 6.00 power meridian. In order to obtain this size and shape of lens we would need a round uncut of at least 64 mm diameter which would allow a wastage of 2 mm all round the shape. Since the 30° meridian is inclined at 60° to the axis meridian, we find, from the tables, that the notional power of the cylinder is + 3.00. Adding this to the sphere the notional power of the lens is + 5.00 along its maximum shape dimension. The meridian of the lens which controls the thickness is the meridian whose sag is greatest over the diameter along the meridian in question.

Figure 80.2

276

In this example our three meridians are 44 mm, 52 mm and 60 mm long. We can find, in the sag tables, which is the greatest sag. *Thus*

    Sag 2.00 at 44? (0.93 mm)
    Sag 5.00 at 60? (4.39 mm) ◀── 4.4 mm
    Sag 6.00 at 52? (3.97 mm)

We find, from the tables, that the greatest sag lies along the $30°$ meridian, sag 5.00 at 60 = 4.39 mm. This meridian, therefore, controls the thickness of the lens. If we required a thin-edge substance of 2 mm, the necessary centre thickness would be about 6.4 mm.

We can now stipulate the thin-edge substance along the + 6.00 meridian of the blank. It is the centre thickness minus sag 6.00 at 64 (6.1 mm), i.e. 0.3 mm. If the thin-edge requirement on the shaped lens had been 1 mm, the centre thickness would be 5.4 mm and the thin edge on the circular blank would be 5.4−6.1 or − 0.7 mm. This minus sign tells us that the blank would begin to knife at a diameter less than 64 mm. Using the sag table we can find the knife-edge diameter for a + 6.00 power by looking along the 6.00 D line for the diameter at which the sag is 5.4 mm. We find, from the table, that the knife-edge diameter is about 60 mm, and we can stipulate in the surfacing data 'knife at 60'.

The purpose of this exercise is to obtain the necessary surfacing data for shaped plus lenses assuming that semi-finished sphere blanks are to be used, and that the sphere power does not exceed + 8.00 D. Information relating to blank selection and minimum thickness is given in previous experiments.

Procedure

(1)   Transpose the prescription, if necessary, to the minus-cylinder transposition.

(2)   Measure the eye of the frame:

    (a)   along the minus-cylinder axis meridian − *Sphere diameter.*

    (b)   at right angles to the minus-cylinder meridian − *Cylinder diameter.*

    (c)   along the longest meridian − *Cutting circle.*

(3)   Measure the angle between the minus-cylinder axis meridian and the longest meridian of the eye and find the notional power of the cylinder along this meridian from the oblique cylinder surface power table. Subtract this value from the sphere to obtain the notional power of the lens along the longest meridian.

(4)   Find:
    (a)   the sag of the sphere at the sphere diameter.
    (b)   the sag of the (sphere + cylinder) at the cylinder diameter.
    (c)   the sag of the notional power at the cutting circle diameter.
(5)   Choose the largest sag found in step 4 and add the minimum edge thickness required from the table of edge thicknesses provided in Experiment 77 to obtain the centre thickness t of the lens.

(6)   Round the centre thickness to the nearest 0.1 mm and check from *Table 77.1* that it lies within the safe range for the sphere power required. IF NOT, DO NOT PROCEED (see Experiment 83).

(7)   Write out the surface powers for the lens, substituting the actual convex surface power given in *Table 77.1* instead of the nominal front surface power. These are the actual surface powers required.

(8)   Find the sag s_1 of the convex surface at the diameter determined in step 5 which controls the thickness of the lens.

(9)   Find the sag s_2 of the notional back surface power (base curve minus notional cylinder) for the same diameter as step 8.

(10)   Find the minimum edge thickness from:

$$e = t - (s_1 - s_2)$$

If this value of e differs by more than 0.1 mm from the minimum edge required add the difference to the edge and centre thicknesses to correct this and again ensure that the centre thickness lies within the safe range given in *Table 77.1*.

(11)   Add 4 mm for wastage to the cutting circle diameter.

(12)   Find the sag s_1 of the convex surface at the new cutting circle diameter.

(13)   Find the sag $s_2 \text{ base}$ of the concave base curve at the new cutting circle diameter.

(14)   Find the minimum edge thickness for the new cutting circle from $e = t - (s_1 - s_2 \text{ base})$. If e is negative find the diameter in mm for which the difference $(s_1 - s_2 \text{ base})$ is the same as t and write 'knife at (the numerical value of this diameter)'.

[*Hint.* Find $s_1 - s_2 \text{ base}$ for the next smaller diameter and repeat until knife-edge diameter is found.]

(15)   Find the sag $s_2 \text{ cross}$ of the concave cross curve at the new cutting circle diameter.

(16)   Find the thick-edge substance at the new cutting circle diameter from:

$$e = t - (s_1 - s_2 \text{ cross})$$

Work through the following examples to confirm the procedure.

278

Examples

(1)   L. + 2.00/+ 4.00 × 90   52 × 44 Quadra

Furthest point on lens periphery 30 mm from SOCP along 150 meridian (see *Figure 80.2*)

+ 6.00/− 4.00 × 180

Sph. diameter = 52 mm

Cyl. diameter = 44 mm

Cutting circle = 60 mm

Angle between 180 and 150 meridian = 30°

Notional power of 4.00 D cylinder at 30° to axis = 1.00 D

Notional power of lens along 150 = 6 − 1 = + 5.00

Sag 6.00 at 52 = 3.97 mm

Sag 2.00 at 44 = 0.93 mm

Sag 5.00 at 60 = 4.39 mm ◄— 4.4 mm

$$t = 4.4 + 1 = 5.4 \text{ mm}$$

Actual surface powers: $\dfrac{+\,9.62}{-\,4.00 \times 90/ \quad 8.00 \times 180}$

Sag 9.62 at 60 = 9.0 mm

Notional back surface power = − 4.00 − 1.00 = − 5.00

Sag 5.00 at 60 = 4.4 mm

$$e = 5.4 − (9.00 − 4.4) = 0.8 \text{ mm}$$

Minimum edge requirement = 1.0 mm. Add 0.2 mm to centre thickness to correct this. t = 5.6 mm

New cutting circle diameter = 64 mm

Sag 9.62 at 64 = 10.4 mm

Sag 4.00 at 64 = 4.0 mm

$$e = 5.6 − (10.4 − 4.0) = − 0.8 \text{ mm on cutting circle}$$

Sag 9.62 at 60 = 9.0 mm |
Sag 4.00 at 60 = 3.5 mm | difference = 5.5 mm

Knife at 60

Sag 8.00 at 64 = 8.4 mm

$$e_{\text{thick}} = 5.6 − (10.4 − 8.4) = 3.6 \text{ mm on cutting circle}$$

(2)   R. $+ 2.50/+ 2.50 \times 180$ 50×40 oval shape

Thin edge = 2.0 mm (metal frame)

$+ 5.00/- 2.50 \times 90$

Sph. diameter = 40 mm   Sag 5.00 at 40 = 1.93 mm

Cyl. diameter = 50 mm   Sag 2.50 at 50 = 1.50 mm

Cutting circle = 50 mm   Sag 2.50 at 50 = 1.50 mm

$t = 1.93 + 2.0 = 3.9$ mm

Actual surface powers: $\dfrac{+ 8.75}{- 4.00 \times 180/- 6.50 \times 90}$

Sag 8.75 at 40 = 3.45 mm

Sag 4.00 at 40 = 1.54 mm

$e = 3.9 - (3.45 - 1.54) = 2.0$ mm

New cutting circle diameter = 54 mm

Sag 8.75 at 54 = 6.45 mm

Sag 4.00 at 54 = 2.82 mm

$e = 3.9 - (6.45 - 2.82) = 0.3$ mm on cutting circle

Sag 6.50 at 54 = 4.67 mm

$e_{thick} = 3.9 - (6.45 - 4.67) = 2.1$ mm on cutting circle

Prescriptions

(1)   R. $+ 1.00/+ 3.50 \times 90$ 50×40 oval shape
(2)   R. $+ 1.00/+ 3.50 \times 180$ 50×40 oval shape
(3)   L. $+ 3.50/+ 2.50 \times 70$ 54×46 sports shape
   Lens measurements: 46 mm along 70
   58 mm along 160

Furthest point on lens periphery 32 mm DOWN and OUT along 130 from SOCP

(4)   L. $- 1.50/+ 4.50 \times 160$ Shape as in (3) above
   2 mm minimum edge for metal

Experiment 81
ASTIGMATIC PRISMATIC LENSES.
SEMI-FINISHED SPHERE BLANKS

Theory

In order to be able to control the thickness of an astigmatic lens which includes a prismatic element, it is necessary to be able to find the effective power of a prism along a meridian other than the base-apex meridian. The effective power of a prism along a meridian inclined at an angle θ to the base-apex meridian is given by

$$P_\theta = P \cos \theta$$

At 90° to the base-apex direction the effective power of the prism is zero.

Table 81.1 has been compiled from this relationship and avoids the need for calculation other than simple addition.

TABLE 81.1. EFFECTIVE PRISM POWER

Prism power	Angle between base-apex direction and oblique meridian							
	10	20	30	40	50	60	70	80
$0.12^\triangle$	$0.12^\triangle$	0.12	0.12	0.12	0.12	–	–	–
$0.25^\triangle$	$0.25^\triangle$	0.25	0.25	0.25	0.12	0.12	0.12	–
$0.50^\triangle$	$0.50^\triangle$	0.50	0.37	0.37	0.37	0.25	0.12	0.12
$1.0^\triangle$	$1.0^\triangle$	1.0	0.87	0.75	0.62	0.50	0.37	0.12
$2.0^\triangle$	$2.0^\triangle$	1.87	1.75	1.5	1.25	1.0	0.75	0.37
$3.0^\triangle$	$3.0^\triangle$	2.87	2.62	2.25	1.87	1.5	1.0	0.50
$4.0^\triangle$	$4.0^\triangle$	3.75	3.5	3.12	2.5	2.0	1.37	0.75
$5.0^\triangle$	$4.87^\triangle$	4.75	4.37	3.87	3.25	2.5	1.75	0.87
$6.0^\triangle$	$5.87^\triangle$	5.75	5.25	4.62	3.87	3.0	2.0	1.0
$7.0^\triangle$	$6.87^\triangle$	6.62	6.0	5.37	4.5	3.5	2.37	1.25
$8.0^\triangle$	$7.87^\triangle$	7.5	6.87	6.12	5.12	4.0	2.75	1.37

The prisms have been rounded to the nearest $0.12^{\triangle}$.

From *Table 81.1*, the effective power of a $1.75^{\triangle}$ prism at 30° to the base-apex direction is seen to be $1.5^{\triangle}$ when rounded to the nearest $0.12^{\triangle}$.

In the following theory the astigmatic prescription is assumed to have been written in its minus-cylinder transposition.

Centre thickness of minus lenses

As with spherical minus lenses which incorporate prism, the centre thickness of the lens must be increased to allow for the prism by the smaller of the two quantities:

(a) Half the prism thickness difference at the blank diameter

(b) $- P^2/10F_{\theta}$ where P is the total prism power and F_{θ} represents the notional power of the lens along the base-apex direction.

Centre thickness of plus lenses

Consider the specification $+ 4.00$ D $\times$ 90 $\bigcirc$ $6^{\triangle}$ base 240 which is to be produced as a 60 mm round uncut with a minimum edge thickness of 1.5 mm. We can imagine that the specification is obtained by combining a knife-edge $+ 4.00$ DC $\times$ 90 with a knife-edge $6^{\triangle}$ prism. Considering only the $+ 4.00$ D cylinder it will have zero edge thickness at the extremities of the 180 meridian, the edge thickness increasing to a maximum along the 90 meridian. Considering only the $6^{\triangle}$ prism base 240, the edge thickness will be zero at 60, increasing to a maximum at 240. When the two elements are combined it is found that the edge thickness decreases between the thinnest point on the cylinder and the thinnest point of the prism. In this example the thinnest point on the edge of the combination is found to lie along 20°. Since the edge substance at this point is the minimum and controls the thickness of the lens it is necessary to be able to locate the point. This can be accomplished by the following construction:

Draw a base line AB to represent the minus-cylinder axis direction. It is convenient to draw AB along the 180 meridian, and of length 10 units.

Construct a perpendicular through B.

Calculate the quantity 200P/dF where P is the power of the prism, d is the uncut diameter and F the power of the cylinder, and construct a line of this length along the acute angle between the prism apex and the minus-cylinder axis meridian BC.

Adjust a ruler so that it passes through point C and so that the distance between the base line and the point D, where the ruler meets the perpendicular from B, is exactly 10 units. The angle DEB then represents the angle between the minus-cylinder axis and the thinnest point on the edge of the lens.

In our example, + 4.00 DC × 90 ◯ 6△ base 240,

$$\frac{200P}{dF} = \frac{200 \times 6}{60 \times 4} = 5 \, (BC)$$

The angle between the prism apex and the minus-cylinder axis is 60° (see *Figure 81.1*). By measurement, angle DEB = 20°.

Figure 81.1

We can now consider how the prism and the cylinder contribute towards the thickness at this point. Since the prism is supposed to be knife-edged the centre thickness of the lens must include half the prism thickness difference at the uncut diameter. The thickness difference for a 6△ prism at 30 mm is found, from the thickness difference table, to be 3.42 mm. The effective prism power along the 20 meridian, at 40° to the base apex direction, is 4.62△ and half the thickness difference for this prism at the uncut diameter is 2.65 mm. The prism is therefore contributing (3.42 − 2.65) = 0.77 mm at this point on the edge.

The notional power of the cylinder along the 20° meridian is + 3.50, from the tables. Assuming the cylinder to be knife-edged and plano-convex in form, the contribution from the cylinder is sag 4.00 at 60 − sag 3.50 at 60, which does not differ much from sag 0.50 at 60, or 0.43 mm. The total thickness at the thinnest point on the edge is therefore 0.77 + 0.43 = 1.2 mm. Since we require a minimum edge of 1.5 mm we must increase the centre thickness by 0.3 mm to provide this. The edge thickness along the minus-cylinder axis can now be determined. The effective power of the prism along 180, inclined at

$60°$ to the base-apex direction of the prism, is $2^\triangle$. The increase in centre thickness necessitated by the prism has already been determined as 3.42 mm. We must add 0.3 mm to this value to obtain the required thin edge, 1.5 mm, at point C. Hence the increase in centre thickness is 3.72 mm. Along the 180 meridian the thinner edge of the lens must be 3.72 minus the thickness difference of a $2^\triangle$ prism at 30 mm, i.e. $3.72 - 1.15 = 2.57$ or 2.6 mm.

At the opposite end of the 180 meridian the edge thickness is 3.72 plus the thickness difference of a $2^\triangle$ prism at 30 mm, i.e. $3.72 + 1.15 = 4.87$ or 4.9 mm.

The purpose of this exercise is to find the surface powers, centre and edge thicknesses of round astigmatic lenses which incorporate prisms assuming that semi-finished sphere blanks are to be used. The procedure outlined below should enable the thin-edge substance to lie within 0.1 mm of the required value.

Procedure

(1)   Compound the prism, if necessary, into a single resultant effect, rounding the resultant to the nearest $0.12^\triangle$ if up to $2^\triangle$ or to the nearest $0.25^\triangle$ if over $2^\triangle$.

(2)   Find the thickness difference g of the prism at the blank diameter from the thickness difference table.

(3)   Transpose the prescription, if necessary, to the minus-cylinder transposition. If the sphere is negative go to step 4.

If the sphere is positive or zero go to step 12.

(4)   Find the notional power of the lens along the base-apex direction, F_θ, by adding the notional power of the cylinder, read from the oblique surface power table, to the sphere.

(5)   Compute the value $- P^2/10F\theta$. Compare this value with half the thickness difference obtained in step 2. The smaller of these two quantities must be added to the centre thickness of the lens selected from the table in Experiment 74 to find the geometric centre thickness t. Round the centre thickness to the nearest 0.1mm.

(6)   Write out the surface powers of the lens substituting the actual convex surface power given in *Table 74.2 or Table 77.1*.

(7)   Find the sag s_1 of the convex surface at the specified diameter from the sag table.

(8)   Find the notional back surface power along the base-apex direction by adding the notional cylinder power, found in step 4, to the base curve.

(9)   Find the sag s_2 of the notional back surface power at the specified diameter from the sag tables.

(10) Find the thin-edge substance along the base-apex direction from $e_{thin} = s_2 - s_1 - g/2 + t$ where $g/2$ is half the prism thickness difference found in step 2 and t is the geometric centre thickness found in step 5.

(11) Find the thick-edge substance along the base-apex direction by adding the thickness difference found in step 2 to the thin-edge substance.

This completes the procedure for minus lenses.

(12) Compute the quantity 200P/dF and complete the graphical construction outlined in the theory above to locate the position of the thinnest point on the edge of the circular blank with respect to the minus-cylinder axis.

(13) Find the effective prism power along the meridian found in step 12 from *Table 81.1*.

(14) Find half the thickness difference of the effective prism power at the blank diameter, $g_\theta/2$, from the thickness difference table and subtract this value from half the thickness difference obtained in step 2.

(15) Find the notional power of the cylinder along the meridian found in step 12 from the oblique surface power table.

(16) Find the sag of the notional cylinder power at the blank diameter and add it to the value obtained in step 14. Compare this result with the edge substance recommended for the lens in Experiment 77 and note any difference. The centre thickness of the lens must be adjusted by this difference in step 18.

(17) Find the sag of the sphere at the blank diameter and add half the thickness difference of the prism obtained in step 2.

(18) Adjust the value obtained in the previous step by the difference found in step 16 to obtain the centre thickness of the lens, t. Check from *Table 77.1* that the centre thickness lies within the safe range for the sphere power required. IF NOT, DO NOT PROCEED.

(19) Write out the surface powers of the lens substituting the actual convex surface power given in Experiment 77 instead of the nominal front surface power. These are the actual surface powers required.

(20) Find the sag s_1 of the convex surface at the specified diameter from the sag tables.

(21) Find the notional back surface power along the thin-edge meridian by adding the notional cylinder power found in step 15 to the base curve.

(22) Find the sag s_2 of the notional back surface power at the blank diameter, from the sag tables.

(23) Find the thin-edge substance from $e = t - (s_1 - s_2) - g\theta/2$. If this value of e differs by more than 0.1 mm from the required value, add the difference to the edge and centre thicknesses to correct this and again ensure that the centre thickness lies within the safe range given for the compensated surface power.

(24) Find the thickness at the opposite edge of the thin-edge meridian by adding the total thickness difference of the effective prism power at the blank diameter (found in step 14) i.e.

$$e_{thick} = e_{thin} + g_\theta.$$

Work through the following examples to confirm the procedure.

Examples

(1) $- 4.00/- 2.00 \times 180$ ◯ $2^\triangle$ base IN   60 mm blank

Thickness difference of $2^\triangle$ prism at 60 mm = 2.3 mm

Power of lens along 180 = $- 4.00$

$- P^2/10F\theta = 4/40 = 0.1$ mm, which is smaller than half the prism thickness difference, so that the centre thickness $t = 1.2 + 0.1 = 1.3$ mm.

Surface powers: $\dfrac{+ 4.00}{- 8.00 \times 90/- 10.00 \times 180}$

Sag 4.00 at 60 = 3.5 mm

Power of back surface along 180 = $- 8.00$

Sag 8.00 at 60 = 7.3 mm

Along base-apex direction,

$$e_{thin} = 7.3 - 3.5 - 1.2 + 1.3 = 3.9 \text{ mm}$$

$$e_{thick} = 3.9 + 2.3 = 6.2 \text{ mm}$$

(2) $- 1.00/- 4.00 \times 30$ ◯ $4^\triangle$ IN   54 mm blank

Thickness difference of $4^\triangle$ prism at 54 = 4.1 mm

Power of lens along 180 = $- 2.00$

$- P^2/10F\theta = 16/20 = 0.8$ mm which is smaller than half the prism thickness difference so that the centre thickness $t = 1.8 + 0.8 = 2.6$ mm.

Surface powers: $\dfrac{+ 5.94}{- 7.00 \times 120/- 11.00 \times 30}$

Sag 5.94 at 54 = 4.2 mm (estimated)

Power of back surface along 180 = − 8.00

Sag 8.00 at 54 = 5.8 mm

Along base-apex direction

$$e_{thin} = 5.8 - 4.2 - 2 + 2.6 = 2.2 \text{ mm}$$

$$e_{thick} = 2.2 + 4.1 = 6.3 \text{ mm}$$

(3)   + 5.00/− 4.00 × 180 $\bigcirc$ 5$^\triangle$ base 240   50 mm blank

Thickness difference of 5$^\triangle$ prism at 50 = 4.76 mm

The graphical construction is exactly the same as the one shown on page 283, from which the minimum edge substance lies along the 20 meridian.

The effective power of the prism along 20, inclined at 40° to the base-apex direction = 3.87$^\triangle$.

Half the thickness difference of 3.87$^\triangle$ at 50 mm = 1.85. Subtracting this from 4.76/2 gives 0.5 mm.

The notional power of the cylinder along 20 = 0.47

Sag 0.47 at 50 = 0.3 mm

Adding 0.5 mm from above gives an edge thickness of 0.8 mm. Since we require a thin edge of 1.0 mm we must increase the centre thickness by 0.2 mm.

Sag 5.00 at 50 = 3.03 mm. Adding half the thickness difference of the 5$^\triangle$ prism, 4.76/2 mm, gives 5.4 mm. This value must be increased by 0.2 mm to provide a thin-edge substance of 1 mm, so that the centre thickness t_1 = 5.6 mm.

Surface powers: $\dfrac{+ 8.75}{- 4.00 \times 90/- 8.00 \times 180}$

Sag 8.75 at 50 = 5.48 mm

The notional back surface power along 20 = − 4.50

Sag 4.50 at 50 = 2.72 mm

Along the 20 meridian,

$$e_{thin} = 5.6 - (5.48 - 2.72) - 1.85 = 1.0 \text{ mm}$$

$$e_{thick} = 1.0 + 3.7 = 4.7 \text{ mm}$$

Prescriptions

(1) R. − 2.00/− 4.00 × 90 ◯ 3△ base UP   60 mm blank
(2) L. − 2.00/+ 4.00 × 135 ◯ 3△ base IN   60 mm blank
(3) R. + 2.00/+ 4.00 × 90 ◯ 4△ base UP   52 mm blank
(4) R. + 2.00/+ 4.00 × 90 ◯ 4△ base IN   52 mm blank
(5) R. + 2.00/+ 4.00 × 90 ◯ 4△ base UP at 60   52 mm blank

Experiment 82
PRISM-TO-CUT

Theory

It is often necessary to produce an uncut lens with the optical centre displaced from the geometric centre. This is achieved by incorporating prism in the lens. In general, it is necessary to find the prismatic effect at the point to which the optical centre is to be shifted, assuming that the optical centre lies at the geometric centre of the lens, and then to incorporate a neutralising prism which will shift the optical centre to the desired position.

For spherical lenses and astigmatic lenses where the decentration coincides with a principal meridian of the lens, the amount of prism required can be found from the simple relationship $P = cF/10$, where c is the desired decentration in millimetres and F the power of the lens along the meridian of decentration.

When the direction of decentration does not coincide with a principal meridian of the lens it is necessary to use a graphical construction to determine the prismatic effect at the point in question. Prism-to-cut must be added to any prescribed prism. When the amount of prism has been determined, together with the base direction, the centre thickness of the lens needs to be increased to allow for the prism. For plus uncut lenses the thickness at the geometric centre should be adjusted using the method given in Experiment 81. With minus lenses the increase in thickness at the geometric centre should be determined by the *smaller* of the two quantities:

(a) Half the thickness difference of the prism at the diameter of the lens.

(b) $- P^2/10F_\theta$ (mm) where P is the amount of prism, and F_θ is the notional power of the lens along the base-apex direction of the prism.

The method for finding the prismatic effect at the point to which the optical centre must be shifted has been explained in Experiment 42, and the method should be revised before proceeding with this experiment.

The purpose of this exercise is to determine the prism necessary to place the optical centre in the required position and to complete the lens specifications for surfacing using semi-finished sphere blanks.

Procedure

(1)   Use the methods detailed in Experiment 42 to determine the prismatic effect at the point to which the optical centre is to be moved.

(2)   Compound the prism into a single resultant effect (see Experiment 40) and reverse the base direction to obtain the necessary prism-to-cut.

(3)   Add any prescribed prism to the prism-to-cut, compounding again, if necessary, to obtain the total prism required on the lens.

(4)   If the lens is spherical, follow the procedure given in Experiment 79. If the lens is astigmatic, follow the procedure given in Experiment 81.

Work through the following examples to obtain surfacing data for the specifications given. Assume that semi-finished sphere blanks are to be used. The relevant details for blank selection and minimum thickness are given in Experiments 74 and 77.

Examples

(1)   R − 4.00 DS dec 5 mm in 52 mm blank

The prismatic effect at a point 5 mm in from the optical centre of a − 4.00 sphere is $2^\triangle$ base IN.

The necessary prism-to-cut is $2^\triangle$ base OUT. The thickness difference of a $2^\triangle$ prism at 52 mm diameter is 2.0 mm; half this value is 1.0 mm.

− $P^2/10F$ = 0.1 mm, and since this is smaller than half the thickness difference, it is the amount which must be added to the centre thickness in order to accommodate the prism.

Hence t = 1.2 + 0.1 = 1.3 mm

Surface powers: $\dfrac{+\,4.00}{-\,8.00}$

Sag 4.00 at 52 = 2.6 mm

Sag 8.00 at 52 = 5.4 mm

$$e_{thin} = s_2 - s_1 - \frac{g}{2} + t \qquad \text{(From Experiment 81)}$$

$$= 5.4 - 2.6 - 1.0 + 1.3 = 3.1 \text{ mm}$$

$$e_{thick} = 3.1 + 2.0 = 5.1 \text{ mm}$$

(2)   L. $- 3.00/- 2.00 \times 135$ ◯ $1^\triangle$ base UP dec 6 mm in 54 blank

The prismatic effect at a point 6 mm in (ignoring the $1^\triangle$ UP) from the optical centre of this lens is $0.6^\triangle$ base DOWN and $2.4^\triangle$ base IN. In order to neutralize this we must work $0.6^\triangle$ base UP and $2.4^\triangle$ base OUT. Adding the prescribed prism we must work a total of $1.6^\triangle$ UP and $2.4^\triangle$ OUT $\equiv 2.88^\triangle$ base UP and OUT at $33°41'$ (say $3^\triangle$ base 35). The thickness difference of a $3^\triangle$ prism at 54 mm is 3.1 mm. Half this value is 1.5 mm.

The notional power of the cylinder along $35°$ (at $80°$ to the axis direction) is $- 1.94$ D. The notional power of the lens along 35 is $- 4.94$. We have $- P^2/10F_\theta = 0.2$ mm and since this is smaller than half the thickness difference of the prism this amount must be added to the centre thickness of the lens.

Hence t = 1.7 mm

The lens surface powers are $\dfrac{+ 4.00}{- 7.00 \text{ DC} \times 45/- 9.00 \text{DC} \times 135}$

The notional power of the back surface along the $35°$ meridian is 8.94

Sag 4.00 at 54 = 2.8 mm.   Sag 8.94 at 54 = 6.6 mm (estimated)

$$e_{thin} = 6.6 - 2.8 - 1.5 + 1.7 = 4.0 \text{ mm}$$

$$e_{thick} = 4.0 + 3.0 = 7.0 \text{ mm}$$

(3)   L. $+ 2.00/+ 3.00 \times 90$ dec 5 mm in 60 mm blank

The prismatic effect at a point 5 mm in from the optical centre is $2.5^\triangle$ base OUT. In order to neutralize this we must work $2.5^\triangle$ IN. The thickness difference of a $2.5^\triangle$ prism at 60 is 2.87 mm.

The prism base coincides with the minus axis meridian and so the minimum edge thickness lies at 180 in standard notation.

The sag of the spherical power of the lens at 60 mm diameter (sag 5.00 at 60) is 4.4 mm, and adding half the thickness difference of the prism and the edge thickness recommended for this power we obtain a centre thickness of 6.8 mm, which lies within the safe range for this type of blank.

The surface powers are $\dfrac{+8.75}{-4.00 \times 90/-7.00 \times 180}$

Sag 8.75 at 60 = 8.1 mm.   Sag 4.00 at 60 = 3.5 mm

$$e_{thin} = t - (s_1 - s_2) - g_\theta/2 \qquad \text{(from Experiment 81)}$$

$$= 6.8 - (8.1 - 3.5) - 1.4 = 0.8 \text{ mm}$$

which is 0.2 mm less than the design value (1.0 mm)

$$e_{thick} = 0.8 + 2.9 = 3.7 \text{ mm}$$

(4)   R. + 2.00/− 4.00 × 30 dec 10 mm in 60 mm blank

The prismatic effect at a point 10 mm in from the optical centre of this lens is $2^\triangle$ base DOWN and OUT at 60. In order to neutralize this we must work $2^\triangle$ base UP and IN at 60.

The thickness difference of $2^\triangle$ prism at 60 = 2.30 mm. 200P/dF = 1.67, and from the graphical construction described in Experiment 81 the thinnest point on the edge is found to lie 5° from the minus-cylinder axis (i.e. at 215°, or DOWN and OUT at 35).

The effective prism power along the 35 meridian is $1.75^\triangle$ and half the thickness difference of this prism at 60 mm diameter is 1.0 mm. The notional power of the cylinder at 5° to its axis is 0.03 D and so the sag of the cylinder can be ignored.

The sag of the sphere at the blank diameter (sag 2.00 at 60) is 1.73 mm, and adding the thickness difference of a $2^\triangle$ prism at 30 gives 2.9 mm.

The recommended edge thickness for this lens is 1.6 mm. The prism will contribute 0.2 mm towards this (2.3/2−1.0), so the centre thickness must be increased by 1.4 mm to provide a minimum edge thickness (at 215°) of 1.6 mm. Hence the centre thickness t = 4.3 mm, which lies within the safe range for this power.

The surface powers are $\dfrac{+6.90}{-5.00 \times 120/-9.00 \times 30}$

$$e_{thin} = t - (\text{sag } 6.90 \text{ at } 60 - \text{sag } 5.00 \text{ at } 60) - 1.0\,(g_\theta/2)$$

$$= 4.3 - (6.2 - 4.4) - 1.0 = 1.5 \text{ mm}$$

$$e_{thick} = 1.5 + 2.0 = 3.5 \text{ mm}$$

Prescriptions

(1) R. − 2.50 dec 6 mm in   56 mm blank

(2) L. + 4.00/+ 2.00 × 90 ◯   1△ base UP dec 5 mm in
                                                     52 mm blank

(3) R. + 2.00/+ 3.00 × 60 dec 4 mm in   54 mm blank

(4) L. − 2.00/+ 4.00 × 135 dec 5 mm in   60 mm blank

(5) R. + 1.50/+ 2.50 × 30 ◯   1△ base DOWN dec 5 mm in
                                                       58 mm blank

Experiment 83
PLUS LENSES. BACK SURFACE
COMPENSATION. SEMI-FINISHED
SPHERE BLANKS

Theory

In previous exercises we have assumed that the arbitrary compensation which is provided by the blank manufacturer on the convex surface of a semi-finished sphere blank is sufficient to produce the correct back vertex power providing the lens thickness does not fall outside a specific range. For example a blank whose nominal front surface power is + 8.00 but has actually been worked with a + 7.80 curve can be used for the thickness range 3.5 to 6.3 mm without introducing an error greater than ± 0.06 D in the back vertex power when the back surface powers are obtained by nominal transposition from the original prescription. If the centre thickness lies outside this range, however, the compensation on the front surface is either too great or too small for the thickness and further compensation must be provided on the back surface.

When the finished centre thickness is less than the minimum value of the safe range then the back surface power must be less minus than the nominal back curve. When the centre thickness is greater than the maximum value of the safe range then the back surface power must be more minus than the nominal back curve.

Consider the prescription + 4.00/− 1.50 × 180 which is to be made (i) 40 mm round with a thin-edge substance of 1.2 mm; (ii) 70 mm round with a thin-edge substance of 2.00 mm. Using the method outlined in Experiment 77 the estimated centre thickness in case (i) would be:

$$\text{sag } 4.00 \text{ at } 40 + 1.2 = 2.70 \text{ mm}$$

which is less than the minimum thickness in the safe range for this power.

If we try to make this lens with the curves obtained by nominal transposition,

$$\frac{+7.80}{-4.00 \times 90/-5.50 \times 180}$$

the actual power of the finished lens would be (using the formulae given in Experiment 51): $+3.91/-1.50 \times 180$ and we find that the sphere is 0.09 D weak. This exceeds the tolerance permitted for this power. Clearly the back surface must be weaker. Assuming that the tool power interval is 0.12 we can work the back surface $-3.87 \times 90/-5.37 \times 180$, which is now acceptable.

In case (ii) the estimated centre thickness would be

$$\text{sag } 4.00 \text{ at } 70 + 2 = 6.8 \text{ mm}$$

which exceeds the maximum thickness in the safe range. If the lens is made with a back surface power of $-4.00 \times 90/-5.50 \times 180$ the actual power of the finished lens would be $+4.08/-1.50 \times 180$ and we find the sphere is $+0.08$ strong. To correct this the back surface power must be increased. If we use the tool $-4.12 \times 90/-5.62 \times 180$ the power of the finished lens would be $+3.96/-1.50 \times 180$ and the error is smaller than the stipulated tolerance.

The procedure is summarised in *Table 83.1*, which shows the additional back surface compensation required for a typical series of semi-finished sphere blanks.

The column headed *Exact centre thickness* gives the centre thickness for which the compensation on the front surface is exactly correct. The column headed *Nominal centre thickness* gives the safe range of centre thicknesses over which the back surface power can be found by nominal transposition. The column headed $+0.12$ gives the range of centre thicknesses for which the back surface power must be weakened by $+0.12$ in order to provide the necessary additional compensation. The column headed -0.12 gives the range of centre thicknesses for which the back surface power must be increased by -0.12 to provide the additional compensation.

The purpose of this exercise is to use the table in conjunction with the table of sags to determine the surface powers, centre and edge thicknesses of plus uncut lenses assuming that semi-finished sphere blanks are to be used.

TABLE 83.1

Nominal base	Exact base	Exact	Centre thickness ranges (mm)			Error	To work powers
			Nominal	+ 0.12	– 0.12		
+ 6.00	+ 5.94	2.6	0 – 5.1	–	5.2 – 10.2	± 0.06	Plano to + 1.00
+ 7.00	+ 6.90	3.2	1.3 – 5.0	UP TO 1.2	5.1 – 8.8	± 0.06	+ 1.25 to + 3.00
+ 8.00	+ 7.80	4.9	3.5 – 6.3	UP TO 3.4	6.4 – 9.2	± 0.06	+ 3.25 to + 4.00
+ 9.00	+ 8.75	4.8	2.6 – 7.0	UP TO 2.5	7.1 – 9.4	± 0.12	+ 4.25 to + 5.00
+ 10.00	+ 9.62	6.0	4.2 – 7.8	2.1 – 4.1	7.9 – 9.7	± 0.12	+ 5.25 to + 6.00
+ 11.50	+ 10.80	8.6	7.2 – 9.9	5.6 – 7.1	10.0 – 11.4	± 0.12	+ 6.25 to + 8.00

PLUS LENSES. BACK SURFACE COMPENSATION. SEMI-FINISHED SPHERE BLANKS

Procedure

(1)   Transpose the prescription, if necessary, to the minus-cylinder transposition.

(2)   Find the sag of the sphere at the specified diameter using the sag tables and round to the nearest 0.1 mm.

(3)   Add the specified edge thickness to the sag found in step 2 to obtain the centre thickness t.

(4)   Use the blank selection table above to determine the form of the lens and whether any further compensation is required for the back surface.

(5)   Write out the surface powers for the lens.

(6)   Find the sags of the convex surface and the concave base curve and hence the thin edge substance from

$$e_{thin} = t - (s_1 - s_{2\ base}).$$

(7)   If e_{thin} differs by more than 0.1 mm from the design value add the difference to the edge and centre thicknesses to correct this and check that the centre thickness remains within the correct range for the compensation.

(8)   If the lens is astigmatic find the sag of the concave cross curve and hence the thick-edge substance from

$$e_{thick} = t - (s_1 - s_{2\ cross}).$$

Work through the following examples to confirm the procedure.

Examples

(1) $+ 8.00/- 2.00 \times 90$ $e_{thin} = 1.0$ mm   50 mm blank

Sag 8.00 at 50 = 5.0 mm

t = 5.0 + 1.0 = 6.0 mm

Surface powers: $\dfrac{+ 10.80}{- 3.37 \times 180/- 5.37 \times 90}$

Sag 10.80 at 50 = 7.0 mm (estimated)

Sag 3.37 at 50 = 2.0 mm (estimated)

$e_{thin} = t - (s_1 - s_{2\ base}) = 6.0 - (7.0 - 2.0) = 1.0$ mm

297

Sag 5.37 at 50 = 3.3 mm (estimated)

$$e_{thick} = t - (s_1 - s_{2 \ cross}) = 6.0 - (7.0 - 3.3) = 2.3 \text{ mm}$$

(2) $+ 5.00 \, \subset \quad 4^{\triangle}$ base IN $e_{thin} = 1.0$ mm   60 mm blank

Sag 5.00 at 60 = 4.4 mm

Since this lens incorporates $4^{\triangle}$ base in prism we must also add the thickness difference of the prism at half the blank diameter to the centre thickness in order to accommodate the prism (see Experiment 79).

Thickness difference of $4^{\triangle}$ prism at 60 = 4.6 mm. Half this value is 2.3 mm

$$t = 4.4 + 2.3 + 1.0 = 7.7 \text{ mm}$$

Surface powers $\dfrac{+ 8.75}{- 4.12}$

Sag 8.75 at 60 = 8.1 mm

Sag 4.12 at 60 = 3.6 mm (estimated)

$$e_{thin} = t - \frac{g}{2} - (s_1 - s_2) = 7.7 - 2.3 - (8.1 - 3.6) = 0.9 \text{ mm}$$

which is within 0.1 mm of the design value.

Prescriptions

(1) $+ 3.00/+ 3.00 \times 60$ $e_{thin} = 1.0$ mm   38 mm round lens

(2) $+ 2.50/+ 3.25 \times 180$ $e_{thin} = 1.0$ mm   70 mm blank

(3) $+ 2.00/+ 6.00 \times 90$ $e_{thin} = 1.2$ mm   50 × 40 oval shape

(4) $+ 2.00/+ 6.00 \times 180$ $e_{thin} = 1.2$ mm   50 × 40 oval shape

(5) $+ 3.50/+ 0.50 \times 90 \, \subset \, 5^{\triangle}$ base IN

$e_{thin} = 1.0$ mm   60 mm blank

Experiment 84
FUSED BIFOCALS

Theory

It was shown in Experiment 57 how the reading addition of a fused bifocal is provided, partly by the difference in front surface powers over the crown and flint glasses, and partly by the contact surface.

We found that the addition A is given by:

$$A = \frac{F_1}{k} - \frac{F_c}{k}$$

where F_1 is the power of the front surface, F_c is the power of the depression curve in air, k is the fused bifocal blank ratio $(n - 1)/(n_s - n)$, n is the refractive index of the crown glass and n_s the refractive index of the segment glass.

Where $n = 1.523$ and $n_s = 1.654$, we find that $k = 4$ (very nearly) and

$$A = \frac{F_1}{4} - \frac{F_c}{4}$$

Thus if the depression curve is -4.00 and the front surface power is $+6.00$, these curves produce an addition:

$$A = \frac{6}{4} - \frac{-4}{4} = +2.50$$

Alternatively, if we have a semi-finished fused bifocal whose front surface power is $+6.00$ and we know that the addition is $+2.00$, then the power of the depression curve is given by:

$$F_c = F_1 - 4\,A = -2.00$$

299

Since the segment is on the front surface of the lens and this side is normally finished by the blank manufacturer, the method for determining the thickness and back surface is precisely the same as that given in Experiments 74 and 77. However, an additional feature of the sequence is that we must ensure that the finished lens substance is thick enough to accommodate the segment without the back curve breaking into the segment. This problem can be deduced from *Figure 57.1*, in which it can be seen that when the centre thickness of the main lens is reduced the back surface will approach the contact surface. A practical guide to the minimum safe centre thickness of the main lens is to ensure that it does not fall below a specific fraction of the reading addition. The fraction depends upon the segment diameter and is given in *Table 84.1* for various common segment diameters. Thus if the segment diameter is 24 mm and the reading addition is + 3.00, the minimum safe centre thickness is $0.6 \times 3 + 0.2 = 2.0$ mm.

TABLE 84.1

Segment diameter	Minimum centre thickness (mm)
22	0.5 A + 0.2
24	0.6 A + 0.2
26	0.7 A + 0.2
28	0.9 A + 0.2
35	1.2 A + 0.2

In the following exercise you should use the blank selection table, *Table 77.1*, in conjunction with a table of sags to determine the surface powers, centre and edge thicknesses of fused bifocal lenses. In each case you must verify that the centre thickness does not fall below the safe value suggested in *Table 84.1*.

Procedure

(1)   Transpose the prescription, if necessary, to the minus-cylinder transposition.

(2)   Compute the minimum safe centre thickness for the lens using *Table 84.1*.

(3)   If the lens is negative follow the procedure given in Experiment 74 but substitute the minimum centre thickness found in (2) if the centre thickness found in Experiment 74 is less than the safe value.

300

(4)   If the lens is positive follow the procedure given in Experiment 77 but substitute the minimum centre thickness found in (2) if the centre thickness found in Experiment 77 is less than the safe value.

Work through the following examples to obtain surfacing data for the specifications given. Assume that the compensation provided on the front segment surface is exactly the same as that provided on semi-finished sphere blanks.

Examples

(1)   R − 5.00 Add 3.00   Fused bifocal

   24 segment   60 mm blank

The minimum safe centre thickness for this lens is 0.6 × 3 + 0.2 = 2.0 mm. This is greater than the value given in Experiment 74 and must be used for this lens.

$$\text{The necessary surface powers are } \frac{+\,4.00}{-\,9.00}$$

$$e_{thin} = \text{sag } 9.00 \text{ at } 60 - \text{sag } 4.00 \text{ at } 60 + t$$

$$= 8.3 - 3.5 + 2 = 6.8 \text{ mm}$$

(2)   L + 4.50/− 1.00 × 90 Add 2.50   Fused bifocal

   22 mm segment   50 mm round blank

The minimum safe centre thickness is 1.5 mm

$$\text{The surface powers are: } \frac{+\,8.75}{-\,4.50 \times 180/-\,5.50 \times 90}$$

The sag of the sphere at 50 mm (sag 4.50 at 50) is 2.7 mm, and adding the thin edge substance from Experiment 77 we obtain a centre thickness of 3.8 mm. This is greater than the minimum safe value and lies within the safe range for nominal transposition.

$$e_{thin} = t - (\text{sag } 8.75 \text{ at } 50 - \text{sag } 4.50 \text{ at } 50)$$

$$= 3.8 - (5.5 - 2.7) = 1.0 \text{ mm}$$

$$e_{thick} = t - (\text{sag } 8.75 \text{ at } 50 - \text{sag } 5.50 \text{ at } 50)$$

$$= 3.8 - (5.5 - 3.4) = 1.7 \text{ mm}$$

Prescriptions

(1)   − 6.00/− 1.00 × 90   Add 2.00 22 segment 60 mm blank
(2)   + 0.50/+ 0.25 × 60   Add 3.00 28 segment 54 mm blank
(3)   + 2.50/+ 1.25 × 180   Add 1.50 24 segment 60 mm blank
(4)   − 1.00/+ 4.00 × 90   Add 2.50 22 segment 56 mm blank
(5)   + 5.00/+ 1.00 × 45   Add 2.00 24 segment 60 mm blank

Experiment 85
SOLID BIFOCALS

Theory

DP Surface. The surface of the distance portion on the segment side.

DP Curve. The power of the DP surface. Solid bifocals are available in four different segment diameters, 22, 30, 38 and 45, and the following DP curves:

Segment diameter mm	Available DP Curves				
22	0.00	− 4.00	− 6.00	− 8.00	− 10.00
30	0.00	− 4.00	− 6.00	− 8.00	
38	0.00	− 4.00	− 6.00	− 8.00	
45	0.00	− 4.00	− 6.00		

Normally, the segment is situated on the back surface of the lens and the front surface must include any cylinder in the form of a plus base toric. Because the base curve and cross curve require different vertex power allowances, there is invariably a tool problem since a very large range of tools is necessary in order to ensure that the power lies within the stipulated tolerance. *Table 85.1* gives details of the DP curves which should be selected for given sphere powers, the prescription, in the case of astigmatic lenses, having first been transposed to plus cylinder form.

303

TABLE 85.1. BLANK SELECTION

DP Curve	To work powers
0.00	over − 10.00
− 10.00	− 4.25 to − 10.00
− 8.00	− 1.75 to − 4.00
− 6.00	+ 2.00 to − 1.50
− 4.00	+ 2.25 to + 8.00
0.00	over + 8.00

The purpose of this exercise is to determine the surface powers, centre thickness and thin edge substance of solid bifocal uncuts using sag tables and vertex power allowance tables. The centre thickness of minus lenses and the edge thickness of plus lenses should be selected from the tables given in Experiments 74 and 77. The procedure outlined below should enable the thin edge substance to lie within 0.2 mm of the value stipulated.

Procedure

(1) Transpose the prescription, if necessary, to the plus-cylinder transposition.

(2) Write out the nominal surface powers of the lens using *Table 85.1* for blank selection.

(3) Transpose the prescription to minus-cylinder form. If the sphere is negative go to step 4. If the sphere is positive or zero go to step 8.

(4) Use the sphere of the minus-cylinder transposition to determine the centre thickness of the lens, t.

(5) Find the sag s_1 of the convex cross curve at the specified diameter.

(6) Find the sag s_2 of the concave DP curve at the specified diameter.

(7) Find the thin edge substance from $e = s_2 - s_1 + t$. This completes the procedure.

(8) Find the sag of the sphere at the specified diameter, and add the thin edge substance stipulated in Experiment 77 for the spherical power. Round the result upwards to the nearest 0.5 mm.

(9) Using the vertex power allowance table find the VPAs for the nominal base curve and cross curve obtained in step 2.

(10) Compensate the front surface by subtracting the VPA (ignoring signs) from the nominal front curves and round the results to the nearest 0.12.

(11) Write out the true surface powers of the lens.

(12) Find the sag s_1 of the convex cross curve at the specified diameter. It will be necessary to estimate 0.12 D curves.

(13) Find the sag s_2 of the concave DP curve at the specified diameter.

(14) Find the thin edge substance from $e = t - (s_1 - s_2)$.

(15) If the edge thickness differs by more than 0.2 mm from the required value adjust the edge and centre thicknesses to correct this.

Work through the following examples to confirm the procedure:

Examples

(1) $- 2.50/- 1.00 \times 180$ Add 2.00

22 segment solid   Blank diameter 60 mm

Plus-cylinder transposition $= - 3.50/+ 1.00 \times 90$

Nominal surface powers: $\dfrac{+ 4.50 \times 180/+ 5.50 \times 90}{- 8.00}$

Centre thickness: 1.5 mm

Sag 5.50 at 60 = 4.86 mm

Sag 8.00 at 60 = 7.29 mm

$e = 7.29 - 4.86 + 1.5 = 3.9$ mm

(2) $+ 2.75/+ 2.00 \times 30$

38 segment solid   Blank diameter 64 mm

Nominal surface powers: $\dfrac{+ 6.75 \times 120/+ 8.75 \times 30}{- 4.00}$

Minus-cylinder transposition $= + 4.75/- 2.00 \times 120$

Sag 4.75 at 64 = 4.75 mm

Centre thickness $= 4.75 + 1.1 = 5.85$ mm

              Round up to 6.0 mm

VPA for $+ 6.75$ at 6.0 mm = 0.17 D

VPA for $+ 8.75$ at 6.0 mm = 0.29 D

305

True surface powers of lens: $\dfrac{+ 6.62 \times 120/+ 8.50 \times 30}{- 4.00}$

Sag 8.50 at 64 = 8.98 mm

Sag 4.00 at 64 = 3.98 mm

e = 6.0 − (8.98 − 3.98) = 1.0 mm

Prescriptions

(1)	− 4.00 Add 1.50 22 seg	60 round blank
(2)	+ 4.00 Add 2.25 45 seg	58 round blank
(3)	− 6.00/− 1.50 × 30 Add 2.00 22 seg	58 round blank
(4)	+ 0.75/+ 0.50 × 90 Add 1.75 38 seg	62 round blank
(5)	+ 7.50/− 0.75 × 80 Add 2.50 45 seg	56 round blank

Experiment 86
EXECUTIVE BIFOCALS

Theory

The Executive bifocal is a solid visible no-jump bifocal with a horizontal dividing line.

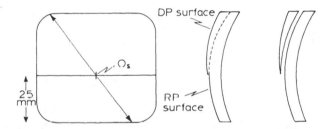

Figure 86.1. The Executive bifocal. Typical blank size = 60 X 56 mm

The segment optical centre lies on the dividing line and it is this feature which gives the design its no-jump property. The thickness of the lens is controlled by the RP curve and the back surface power for, as the diagram above suggests, we may consider the lens as a base element, whose power is the reading prescription, on to which is attached a minus element, the power of which is equal to minus the reading addition. Ideally, the DP surface and RP surface should be tangential at the centre of the ledge but there is usually a step the depth of which can be up to 0.5 mm. We will assume the depth of ridge is 0.3 mm in the following exercise:

The Executive blank is rectangular in shape and in order to specify the thickness with respect to the edge of the blank, it is necessary to know how far the segment centre is from the edge of the lens in each meridian. This information is given in *Table 86.1*. The first figure gives the distance from the segment centre to the edge of the RP and the second figure gives the distance from the segment centre to the edge of the DP.

TABLE 86.1

Meridian	Distance from O_S to lens edge	
	RP	DP
180	30	30
10 or 170	31	31
20 or 160	32	32
30 or 150	35	35
40 or 140	36	39
50 or 130	35	39
60 or 120	30	36
70 or 110	28	33
80 or 100	26	31
90	25	31

The distance optical centre can be positioned anywhere in the DP. In the absence of prescribed prism we will assume that it is to be placed on the dividing line (segment drop = 0 mm). The difference in thickness between this point and the segment optical centre on the RP surface will be taken to be simply the depth of the ridge, 0.3 mm.

Table 86.2 shows a typical range of DP curves for the Executive bifocal and may be used for blank selection. The table also gives the safe thickness ranges for each DP curve.

The column headed *'Exact centre thickness'* gives the centre thickness for which the compensation on the front surface is exactly correct.

The column headed *'Nominal centre thickness'* gives the safe range of centre thicknesses over which the back surface power can be found by nominal transposition.

The column headed + 0.12 gives the range of centre thicknesses for which the back surface power must be weakened by 0.12 in order to provide the necessary additional compensation.

The column headed − 0.12 gives the range of centre thicknesses for which the back surface power must be increased by − 0.12 to provide the additional compensation.

TABLE 86.2

Nominal base	Exact base	Centre thickness ranges, mm				Error	To work powers
		Exact	Nominal	+ 0.12	− 0.12		
+ 3.00	+ 2.96	–	0 – 27.2	–	–	± 0.12	Over − 5.50
+ 4.50	+ 4.44	–	0 – 9.2	–	–	± 0.06	− 5.50 to − 2.25
+ 5.75	+ 5.67	3.7	1.0 – 6.5	Up to 0.9	6.6 – 11.8	± 0.06	− 2.00 to 0.00
+ 6.50	+ 6.41	3.3	1.1 – 5.4	Up to 1.0	5.5 – 9.6	± 0.06	+ 0.25 to + 1.25
+ 7.25	+ 7.15	2.9	1.2 – 4.6	Up to 1.1	4.7 – 8.0	± 0.06	+ 1.50 to + 3.00
+ 8.00	+ 7.89	2.7	1.2 – 4.0	Up to 1.1	4.1 – 6.8	± 0.06	+ 3.25 to + 4.00
+ 9.00	+ 8.88	2.3	0 – 4.5	–	4.6 – 6.9	± 0.12	+ 4.25 to + 6.00

The purpose of this exercise is to use the above tables in conjunction with surfacing tables to determine the surface powers, centre and edge thicknesses of uncut Executive bifocals. The centre thickness of minus lenses and edge thickness of plus lenses should be selected from the tables given in Experiments 74 and 75.

Procedure

(1)   Transpose the prescription, if necessary, to the minus-cylinder transposition.

(2)   Write out the front surface power and the nominal back curves using *Table 86.2* for blank selection (use the sphere from the minus cylinder Rx).

(3)   If the lens is astigmatic note the blank dimensions from *Table 86.1* for the RP and DP along the cylinder axis meridian. If the lens is spherical use the maximum values given (for the 40 or 140 meridians) in *Table 86.1*.

(4)   Add the reading addition to the sphere of the minus-cylinder transposition. If the result is negative go to step 5. If the result is positive go to step 13.

(5)   Use the sphere plus the reading addition obtained in step 4 to determine the centre thickness of the lens and add 0.3 mm to obtain the centre thickness t.

(6)   Write out the actual surface powers of the lens.

(7)   Find the sag $s_1 R$ of the convex RP curve (DP curve + Add) at the RP diameter obtained in step 3.

(8)   Find the sag $s_2 R$ of the concave base curve at the RP diameter.

(9)   Find the thin edge substance on the RP from $e_R = s_2 R - s_1 R + t - 0.3$.

(10)   Find the sag $s_1 D$ of the convex DP curve at the DP diameter obtained in step 3.

(11)   Find the sag $s_2 D$ of the concave base curve at the DP diameter.

(12)   Find the thin edge substance on the DP from $e_D = s_2 D - s_1 D + t$. This completes the procedure for negative lenses.

(13)   Use the sphere plus the reading addition obtained in step 4 to determine the thin edge substance of the lens from *Table 77.2*.

(14)   Find the sag of the sphere plus the reading addition at the RP diameter obtained in step 3 and add 0.3 and the thin-edge substance to obtain the centre thickness t.

(15)   Use the blank selection table (*Table 86.2*) to determine the surface powers of the lens and whether any additional compensation is required for the back surface.

(16)   Write out the surface powers for the lens.

(17) Find the sag $s_1 R$ of the convex RP curve (DP curve + Add) at the RP diameter.

(18) Find the sag $s_2 R$ of the concave base curve at the RP diameter.

(19) Find the thin-edge substance on the RP from
$$e_R = t - (s_1 R - s_2 R) - 0.3.$$

(20) Find the sag $s_1 D$ of the convex DP curve at the DP diameter.

(21) Find the sag $s_2 D$ of the concave base curve at the DP diameter.

(22) Find the thin-edge substance on the DP from
$$e_D = t - (s_1 D - s_2 D).$$

Work through the following examples to confirm the procedure.

Examples

(1) $- 4.00$ Add 2.00   Executive bifocal

Form $= \dfrac{+ 4.44}{- 8.50}$

RP diameter = 2 × 36 = 72 mm   DP diameter = 2 × 39 = 78 mm

Sphere + Add = $- 2.00$

$$t - 1.6 + 0.3 - 1.9 \text{ mm}$$

Actual surface powers: $\dfrac{+ 4.44}{- 8.50}$

RP curve = $+ 6.44$

Sag 6.44 at 72 = 8.4

Sag 8.50 at 72 = 11.6

$$e_R = 11.6 - 8.4 + 1.9 - 0.3 = 4.8 \text{ mm}$$

Sag 4.44 at 78 = 6.6

Sag 8.50 at 78 = 13.9

$$e_D = 13.9 - 6.6 + 1.9 = 9.2 \text{ mm}$$

(2) $- 0.50/- 1.00$ × 60 Add 2.50   Executive bifocal

Form $= \dfrac{+ 5.67}{- 6.25 \times 150/- 7.25 \times 60}$

RP diameter = 2 × 30 = 60 mm

311

DP diameter = 2 × 36 = 72 mm

Sphere + Add = + 2.00

$$e_{thin} = 1.6 \text{ mm}$$

Sag 2.00 at 60 = 1.7 mm

$$t = 1.7 + 0.3 + 1.6 = 3.6 \text{ mm}$$

Actual surface powers: $\dfrac{+ 5.67}{- 6.25 \times 150 / - 7.25 \times 60}$

RP curve = + 8.17

Sag 8.17 at 60 = 7.5 mm

Sag 6.25 at 60 = 5.6 mm

$$e_R = 3.6 - (7.5 - 5.6) - 0.3 = 1.4 \text{ mm}$$

Sag 5.67 at 72 = 7.3 mm

Sag 6.25 at 72 = 8.1 mm

$$e_D = 3.6 - (7.3 - 8.1) = 4.4 \text{ mm}$$

(3)   + 5.00/− 2.00 × 90   Add 1.50   Executive bifocal

Form = $\dfrac{+ 8.88}{- 4.00 \times 180 / - 6.00 \times 90}$

RP diameter = 2 × 25 = 50 mm

DP diameter = 2 × 31 = 62 mm

Sphere + Add = + 6.50

$$e_{thin} = 1.0 \text{ mm}$$

Sag 6.50 at 50 = 4.0 mm

$$t = 4.0 + 1.0 + 0.3 = 5.3 \text{ mm}$$

Actual surface powers = $\dfrac{+ 8.88}{- 4.12 \times 180 / - 6.12 \times 90}$

RP curve = + 10.38

Sag 10.38 at 50 = 6.6 mm

Sag 4.12 at 50 = 2.5 mm

$$e_R = 5.3 - (6.6 - 2.5) - 0.3 = 0.9 \text{ mm}$$

Sag 8.88 at 62 = 8.8 mm

Sag 4.12 at 62 = 3.8 mm

$$e_D = 5.3 - (8.8 - 3.8) = 0.3 \text{ mm}$$

Prescriptions

(1)   + 2.00 Add 2.00
(2)   − 3.00/+ 0.50 × 70 Add 1.25
(3)   + 5.00/− 2.00 × 180 Add 1.50
(4)   − 0.50/− 0.75 × 10 Add 2.50
(5)   + 3.00/+ 1.00 × 120 Add 2.25

Experiment 87
DEEP PLUS FLATS

Theory

High plus prescriptions are often dispensed in plano-convex form with any correction for astigmatism incorporated on the back surface of the lens as a plano-convex or plano-concave cylinder. In order to ensure that the finished glazed lens is no thicker than necessary it is usual to custom design these lenses to the final shape, i.e. to stipulate a specific edge thickness at a specific diameter. This task is greatly simplified by means of tables which give the centre thickness together with the compensated plus curve for various powers and diameters.

Consider the plano-convex lens illustrated in *Figure 87.1*. The centre thickness t is the sum of the thin-edge substance e and the sag of the front convex curve F_1 at the diameter 2y. Since F_1 is unknown at the outset the usual methods for accurate transposition cannot be applied; t and F_1 are interdependent.

Figure 87.1

When surfacing this type of lens it is usual to make the edge thickness e as small as possible. If e = 0 the lens is said to be *knife-edged*. In practice we cannot actually obtain a true knife-edge since the edge would begin to crumble. In order to obtain a specific diameter it will be assumed that an edge thickness of 0.5 mm is sufficiently close to

314

zero to enable the lens to be produced at the stated diameter. The real criterion for the optimum edge thickness is the type of edge which is eventually employed to secure the lens to the frame. For a bevel edge, the edge thickness at the glazing diameter should be about 1 mm and this value should be checked before determining the final centre thickness of the lens.

Consider a + 10.00 D lens which is to be made in plano-convex form and used for the lens shape depicted in *Figure 87.2*. As can be seen from the diagram the instruction has called for a 2 mm inward decentration, and the minimum diameter of a circular uncut which gives a 1 mm allowance for edging is 50 mm. Using tables which give the centre thickness and compensated front curve for 'strong positive lenses of specified diameter and edge thickness' we find that the centre thickness and front curve which will produce + 10.00 at 50 mm diameter with an edge thickness of 0.5 mm are given by t = 6.57 mm, F_1 = + 9.59. Rounding the centre thickness upwards to 6.6 mm and the front curve downwards to + 9.50 produces the data: t = 6.6 mm, F_1 = + 9.50.

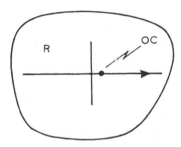

Figure 87.2

We should now check the edge thickness at the glazing diameter of 48 mm. From the sag tables, sag 9.50 at 48 mm diameter = 5.5 mm, and the edge thickness at 48 mm would be t − 5.5 or 1.1 mm, which value is about ideal for the lens.

The following rule should be used for rounding curves and thickness. If we are rounding the front curve *upwards* we must round the thickness *downwards* and when we round the front curve *downwards*, as in this first example, we must round the thickness *upwards*.

Consider now the prescription + 10.00/+ 4.00 × 90. If this was made as a plano-cylinder lens with a true knife-edge all round the lens periphery it would be elliptical in shape. The short diameter of the ellipse would lie along the maximum power meridian (180) and the long diameter lies along the minimum power meridian (90). It is important to check that the *short* diameter will encompass the finished lens shape. Suppose that we had determined that the short diameter necessary to just encompass a given lens shape is 52 mm. Adding a 1.0 mm allowance all round the edge for wastage we want to produce + 10.00/ + 4.00 X 90 at 54 mm with a thin-edge thickness of 0.5 mm.

(A) Minus-cylinder flat

The nominal front curve is + 14.00 DS. From the tables we find that the centre thickness and compensated front curve for + 14.00 at 54 mm diameter are 10.64 mm and + 12.75 D. Rounding the centre thickness to 10.6 mm we have the data:

$$\frac{+ 12.75}{- 4.00 \times 180} \qquad t = 10.6 \text{ mm}$$

At the glazing diameter (52mm) the thin edge will be 10.6 − sag 12.75 at 52 = 10.6 − 9.3 = 1.3 mm.

(B) Plus-cylinder flat

The nominal front curve is + 10.00 DS and the centre thickness must include the sag of a + 4.00 D cylinder, which is not accounted for in the tables. Sag 4.00 at 52 (the glazing diameter) is 2.6 mm. From the tables for strong positive lenses of specified diameter and edge thickness the centre thickness and compensated front curve for + 10.00 at 54 mm are 7.6 mm and + 9.52. Adding the sag of the cylinder we need a final centre thickness of 10.2 mm.

Now using vertex power allowance tables we must confirm that the vertex power allowance is still correct for the increased centre thickness. From the tables the vertex power allowance for a + 10.00 D nominal curve at 10.2 mm thickness is − 0.62 D and the nearest 0.12 tool is + 9.37.

Hence the final surfacing data are:

$$\frac{+ 9.37}{+ 4.00 \times 90} \qquad t = 10.2 \text{ mm}$$

At the glazing diameter (52 mm) the thin edge will be t − sag 9.37 at 52 − sag 4.00 at 52. This equals 10.2 − 6.4 − 2.6 = 1.2 mm.

In the following exercise you should use tables for strong positive lenses of specified diameter and edge thickness in conjunction with sag tables to determine the centre thickness and compensated front surface power for deep plus flat lenses. Assume that astigmatic lenses are to be made in both minus- and plus-cylinder form.

Procedure

(1) Transpose the prescription, if necessary, to the minus-cylinder transposition.

(2) Add 2.0 mm to the glazing diameter given for the lens.

(3) Using the sphere of the minus-cylinder transposition of the prescription as the nominal front curve, find, from the tables, the centre thickness and compensated front curve for the diameter determined in step 2.

(4) Round the compensated front curve to the nearest 0.12 power and the centre thickness to the nearest 0.1 mm.

(5) Find the sag of the compensated front curve at the glazing diameter and subtract from the centre thickness to obtain the thin-edge substance for edging.

(6) If the lens is astigmatic, transpose the prescription to the plus-cylinder form.

(7) Find the sag of the cylinder at the *glazing* diameter, i.e. the diameter given for the prescription.

(8) Use the sphere of the plus-cylinder transposition as the nominal front curve to read from the tables the centre thickness and compensated front curve for this form.

(9) Add the sag of the cylinder found in step 7 to the centre thickness obtained in step 8 to determine the centre thickness for the lens.

(10) Check that the vertex power allowance for the new centre thickness is still sufficient within 0.12 D. If not, reduce the compensated front curve a further 0.12 D and re-check.

(11) Find the sag of the final compensated front curve and the sag of the cylinder at the glazing diameter and subtract both from the centre thickness to obtain the thin edge substance for edging.

Work through the following examples to confirm the procedure.

Examples

(1)   + 12.25 DS glazing diameter: 48 mm

Surfacing diameter = 50 mm

From the tables for strong positive lenses of specified diameter and edge thickness, t = 8.0 mm, F_1 = + 11.51 D.

Hence $\dfrac{+11.50}{\text{Plano}}$ $t = 8.0$ mm

Sag 11.50 at 48 = 6.9 mm, so that the glazing edge thickness is $8.0 - 6.9 = 1.1$ mm.

(2) $+17.00/-3.00 \times 90$ glazing diameter: 54 mm.

Surfacing diameter = 56 mm

From the tables for strong positive lenses, $t = 14.11$ mm, $F_1 = +14.69$ D.

Hence $\dfrac{+14.75}{-3.00 \times 90}$ $t = 14.1$ mm

Sag 14.75 at 54 = 12.5 mm, so that the glazing edge thickness is $14.1 - 12.5 = 1.6$ mm.

The plus-cylinder transposition of this prescription is $+14.00/+3.00 \times 180$.   Sag 3.00 at 54 = 2.1 mm

From the tables for strong positive lenses, $t = 11.45$ mm, $F_1 = 12.67$.

Hence $\dfrac{+12.62}{+3.00 \times 180}$ $t = 11.5 + 2.1 = 13.6$ mm

The vertex power allowance for a nominal $+14.00$ at 13.6 mm thickness is -1.56, i.e. the compensated front curve should be $+12.44$. We must, therefore, reduce the compensated front curve to $+12.50$.

The final form of the lens is:

$$\frac{+12.50}{+3.00 \times 180} \qquad t = 13.6 \text{ mm}$$

Sag 12.50 at 54 = 9.9 mm, so that the glazing edge thickness is $13.6 - 9.9 - 2.1 = 1.6$ mm.

Prescriptions

(1)	$+9.50$ DS	glazing diameter 46 mm
(2)	$+10.25/+0.75 \times 60$	glazing diameter 44 mm
(3)	$+11.50/+3.50 \times 180$	glazing diameter 42 mm
(4)	$+10.75/-1.75 \times 45$	glazing diameter 56 mm
(5)	$+10.00/+4.00 \times 180$	glazing diameter 58 mm

Experiment 88
HIGH REFRACTIVE INDEX GLASS LENSES

Theory

Occasionally a prescription is dispensed in high refractive index glass, e.g. Highlite, whose refractive index is 1.701, in order to obtain thinner lenses. Surfacing laps, however, are calibrated for ophthalmic crown glass of refractive index 1.523, so that the powers which they produce on glasses of other refractive indices are not those marked on the laps.

The radius of curvature of the lap face is 523/F mm where F is the power marked on the lap. The actual power which this radius r imparts on glass of refractive index n is $1000(n - 1)/r$. Thus if a lap marked 10.00 D is used on 1.701 index glass the actual surface power which it will produce can be deduced as follows:

Radius of 10.00 D lap = 523/10 = 52.3 mm
Power of surface on 1.701 index glass = 701/52.3 = 13.40 D

Normally, only minus lenses are made in high refractive index glass since there is a noticeable reduction in edge thickness. Although plus lenses would also be thinner, the reduction in centre thickness is not apparent to the observer. This exercise is limited to the writing of surfacing tickets for minus lenses.

It is assumed that rough blanks of high refractive index glass are available and both the plus and minus surfaces are to be worked with tools calibrated for glass of refractive index 1.523. *Table 88.1* may be used for blank selection, the prescription being taken, when necessary, in minus-cylinder transposition.

TABLE 88.1

1.523 Base	True power on 1.701 glass	To work powers	Centre thickness
+ 3.75	+ 5.00	− 4.00 to − 5.75	1.2 mm
+ 3.00	+ 4.00	− 6.00 to − 7.75	1.0 mm
+ 2.25	+ 3.00	− 8.00 to − 9.50	1.0 mm
+ 1.50	+ 2.00	− 9.75 to − 12.00	1.0 mm
+ 1.00	+ 1.37	− 12.25 to − 14.00	1.0 mm
+ 0.50	+ 0.62	− 14.25 to − 16.00	1.0 mm
0.00	0.00	over − 16.00	1.0 mm

Suppose it is required to produce the lens − 6.00/− 2.00 × 90 in glass of refractive index 1.701. From *Table 88.1* we would choose a + 3.00 D spherical tool to work the front curve. The actual power of the front surface is seen, from the table, to be + 4.00. The back surface power must therefore be − 10.00 × 180/− 12.00 × 90 to obtain the correct prescription. The 1.523 index tools which will produce these curves can be deduced as follows:

The radius of the 10.00 D curve is 701/10 = 70.1 mm. The 1.523 tool which has this radius is 523/70.1 = − 7.46 or − 7.50. This value can be found directly by multiplying the 1.701 curve required by 0.523/0.701 or 0.746. Hence the cross curve power, − 12.00, is produced by the 1.523 index tool marked 12 × 0.746 = − 8.95 or − 9.00.

The form of the lens is:

1.523
curves

$$\frac{+ 3.00 \text{ DS}}{- 7.50 \times 180/- 9.00 \times 90}$$

1.701
powers

$$\frac{+ 4.00 \text{ DS}}{- 10.00 \times 180/- 12.00 \times 90}$$

The actual sphere power which the 1.523 curves have produced can be found by adding the sphere curve and base curve together and multiplying by 0.701/0.523 or 1.34. The actual cylinder power can be found by multiplying the 1.523 cylinder by 1.34. These values should be checked to ensure that the sphere and cylinder lie within the acceptable tolerance range. We find:

Sphere = − 4.50 × 1.34 = − 6.03
Cylinder = − 1.50 × 1.34 = − 2.01

The thin and thick edge substances may be found by reading the sags of the 1.523 curves from the sag tables.

Prescribed prism, or prism-to-cut, must also be converted to 1.523 prism values in order to obtain the correct amounts of prism. The actual prism required may be given, or calculated, as in previous exercises and should be multiplied by 0.746 to find the 1.523 prism value. For example, a $3^{\triangle}$ prism which is to be incorporated in a 1.701 index lens must be ground as 3 × 0.746 or $2.25^{\triangle}$, and the thickness difference of this latter value may be obtained from 1.523 index charts.

Procedure

(1) Transpose the prescription, if necessary, to the minus-cylinder transposition.

(2) Use the Blank Selection (*Table 88.1*) to determine the 1.523 tool for the front surface, its 1.701 index value and the centre thickness for the lens.

(3) If prism or decentration has been prescribed use the method detailed in Experiment 82 to find the single resultant prism and multiply the resultant by 0.746 to obtain the 1.523 equivalent. Find the notional power of the lens along the prism base-apex direction, and the thickness difference g of the prism, and compute the value $- P^2/10F_\theta$. Add the smaller value, $g/2$ or $- P^2/10F_\theta$, to the centre thickness to find the geometric centre thickness.

(4) Using the 1.701 index front curve, write out the surface powers of the lens.

(5) Multiply the base curve and cross curve by 0.746 to obtain the 1.523 index tools necessary to work the back surface, rounding the curves to the nearest 0.12.

(6) Add the 1.523 index sphere curve to the 1.523 index base curve and multiply the result by 1.34 to find the true sphere which will be produced. Check that the sphere lies within the accepted tolerance range for the power.

(7) Multiply the difference between the 1.523 index base curve and the 1.523 index cross curve by 1.34 to find the true cylinder which will be produced. Check that the cylinder lies within the accepted tolerance range.

(8) Find the sag s_1 of the 1.523 index convex sphere curve at the blank diameter.

(9) Find the sag s_2 of the 1.523 index base curve at the blank diameter.

(10) Find the thin edge substance from $e_{thin} = s_2 - s_1 + t$.

(11) If the lens incorporates a prism find the notional back surface power along the base-apex direction by adding the notional cylinder to the base curve.

(12) Find the sag of the notional back surface power from the tables.

(13) Find the thin edge substance along the base-apex direction from $e_{thin} = s_2 - s_1 - g/2 + t$.

(14) Find the thick edge substance along the base-apex direction by adding the thickness difference g to the result obtained in step 13.

Work through the following examples to confirm the procedure.

Examples

(1) $- 8.00$ DS dec 5 mm IN   60 mm blank

1.523 index front curve = $+ 2.25$

1.701 index front curve = $+ 3.00$ $t = 1$ mm

Prism-to-cut = $4^\triangle$ OUT

1.523 prism = $3^\triangle$ OUT

$- P^2/10F_\theta = 0.11$ mm

$g = 3.4$ mm $g/2 = 1.7$ mm

Since 0.11 mm is the smaller, this must be added to the centre thickness, hence t = 1.1 mm

1.701 index curves = $\dfrac{+ 3.00}{- 11.00}$

1.523 index back curve = $- 11.00 \times 0.746 = - 8.25$

1.523 index curves = $\dfrac{+ 2.25}{- 8.25}$

Actual power produced = $- 6.00 \times 1.34 = - 8.04$

Sag 2.25 at 60 = 1.9 mm

Sag 8.25 at 60 = 7.5 mm

$$e_{thin} = 7.5 - 1.9 - 1.7 + 1.1 = 5.0 \text{ mm}$$
$$e_{thick} = 5.0 + 3.4 = 8.4 \text{ mm}$$

(2) $- 10.50/- 1.50 \times 30$ 52 mm blank

1.523 index front curve = $+ 1.50$

1.701 index front curve = $+ 2.00$ $t = 1.0$ mm

$$1.701 \text{ index curves} = \frac{+ 2.00}{- 12.50 \times 120/- 14.00 \times 30}$$

1.523 index base curve = $- 12.50 \times 0.746 = - 9.37$

1.523 index cross curve = $- 14.00 \times 0.746 = - 10.50$

$$1.523 \text{ index curves: } \frac{+ 1.50}{- 9.37 \times 120/- 10.50 \times 30}$$

Actual sphere power produced = $- 7.87 \times 1.34 = - 10.55$

Actual cylinder power produced = $- 1.12 \times 1.34 = - 1.50$

Sag 1.50 at 52 = 1.0 mm

Sag 9.37 at 52 = 6.4 mm

$$e_{thin} = 6.4 - 1.0 + 1.0 = 6.4 \text{ mm}$$

Prescriptions

(1)	$- 20.00$	50 mm blank
(2)	$- 7.25/+ 1.75 \times 90$	58 mm blank
(3)	$- 6.50/- 0.50 \times 45 \circlearrowright \ 2^{\triangle}$ IN	60 mm blank
(4)	$- 7.50/- 3.00 \times 30$ dec 4 mm IN	60 mm blank
(5)	$- 12.00/+ 2.25 \times 180$	52 mm blank

Experiment 89
THE AIR CELL

Theory

The air cell consists essentially of a parallel-sided block of glass enclosing air and immersed in a liquid whose refractive index we wish to determine. The rotation of the cell about a vertical axis can be measured on a circular scale.

Figure 89.1 shows the air cell immersed in a liquid of refractive index n_L. Let the glass have refractive index n_g.

Figure 89.1

The incident ray AB makes an angle $\theta/2$ with the normal, and is refracted as ray BC into the glass block. Ray BC is incident at the glass-air interface at the critical angle for the glass/air interface and emerges into the air film along the direction CD. Hence $\theta/2$ is the critical angle for ray AB in liquid of refractive index n_L since it cannot pass through the air cell. Let us apply the law of refraction at each surface. At the point B:

$$n_L \sin\frac{\theta}{2} = n_g \sin i_c$$

(i_c is the critical angle for glass to air)

At the point C:

$$n_g \sin i_c = \sin 90°$$

Combining these two equations, we have:

$$n_L \sin\frac{\theta}{2} = \sin 90° = 1$$

Therefore

$$n_L = 1/\sin\frac{\theta}{2} = \operatorname{cosec}\frac{\theta}{2}$$

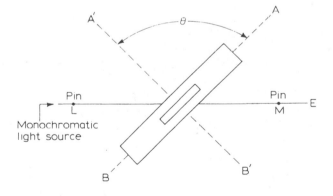

Figure 89.2

Procedure

Figure 89.2 shows the cell in a position AB with an eye at E in line with pins L and M and a shadow is seen covering half the cell.

The reading on the circular scale is recorded. The air cell is rotated through an angle θ into the position A'B', when a shadow is seen covering the other half of the air cell. The new reading on the circular scale is recorded, and the difference between the two readings is θ. Then θ is twice the critical angle for light passing from liquid to air and the refractive index of the liquid is cosec $\theta/2$.

Repeat for various positions of AB, obtaining corresponding positions A'B'.

Calculate the critical angle and the refractive index of water and other liquids provided.

Experiment 90
MINIMUM DEVIATION OF A PRISM

Theory

In *Figure 90.1* ray GE makes an angle of incidence i_1 with the normal EF. After refraction at the first face of the prism it makes an angle of refraction i'_1. At the second face AC of the prism the angles of incidence and refraction are i_2 and i'_2 respectively.

Figure 90.1

Since EF is normal to AB and FD is normal to AC, the quadrilateral AEFD is cyclic; hence angle EFD = $180° - A$, where A is the apical angle of the prism.

The incident ray undergoes deviation d_1 at the first face and deviation d_2 at the second face. Hence the total deviation $D = d_1 + d_2$.

From *Figure 90.1*

$$d_1 = i_1 - i'_1 \qquad \qquad \dots \ (1)$$

$$d_2 = i'_2 - i_2 \qquad \qquad \dots \ (2)$$

From equations (1) and (2)

$$D = (i_1 + i'_2) - (i'_1 + i_2) \qquad \ldots (3)$$

In triangle EFD it has already been shown that $EFD = 180° - A$

Hence
$$i'_1 + i_2 = A \qquad \ldots (4)$$

From equations (3) and (4)

$$D = i_1 + i'_2 - A \qquad \ldots (5)$$

It can be shown that the deviation D is a minimum when the path of light is symmetrical through the prism. Hence this minimum occurs when

$$i'_1 = i_2 \qquad \ldots (6)$$

and
$$i_1 = i'_2 \qquad \ldots (7)$$

From equations (4) and (6)

$$2i'_1 = A \text{ or } i'_1 = \frac{A}{2} \qquad \ldots (8)$$

and from equations (5) and (7)

$$D = 2i_1 - A \text{ or } i_1 = \frac{A + D}{2} \qquad \ldots (9)$$

Let n be the refractive index of the prism; then from the law of refraction

$$\sin i_1 = n \sin i'_1 \qquad \ldots (10)$$

From equations (8), (9) and (10)

$$n = \frac{\sin \dfrac{A + D}{2}}{\sin \dfrac{A}{2}} \qquad \ldots (11)$$

when D is the angle of minimum deviation.

Apparatus

Prism, drawing board, paper and pins.

Procedure

(1) Place the prism on a sheet of paper and outline its position.

328

Place the pins at G and E (see *Figure 90.1*). Look through the prism and place pins at D and H so that they appear in line with pins G and E.

(2) Remove the prism and measure angles i_1 and i'_2. (Since the path of light is reversible each observation will give rise to two values for the angle of incidence.) Hence measure the deviation D.

Measure the apical angle A of the prism and verify that $D = i_1 + i'_2 - A$.

(3) Repeat at least six times with different values of i_1.

(4) Draw a graph plotting i_1, horizontally and D vertically connecting the points by a smooth curve. You should obtain a graph of the form WVW' as shown in *Figure 90.2*. Draw a tangent to the lowest point V of the curve. The tangent will intersect the vertical axis at the point where D will be a minimum. Substitute this value in equation (11) and hence calculate the refractive index of the prism.

Figure 90.2. Curve WVW' shows the variation of D with angle of incidence i_1. It can be shown that the mid-points of all chords parallel to WYW' lie on the line $2x = A + y$, which passes through V corresponding to the minimum value of D. The intercept on the x axis of line YV is half the apical angle. Hence the intercept has the value $30°$ as shown when the apical angle of the prism is $60°$

(5) Draw the chord WW' parallel to the x axis. Obtain the mid-point Y. Draw the line YV until it intercepts the x axis. Measure the gradient of the graph, and obtain the value of the intercept on the x axis. The gradient should have a value of 2 and the intercept should have the value A/2.

Experiment 91
THE SPECTROMETER: APICAL ANGLE OF A PRISM; REFRACTIVE INDEX BY THE METHOD OF MINIMUM DEVIATION

Theory and Procedure

Setting up the spectrometer

The following steps must be carried out in all spectrometer experiments:

(1) Observe the cross-wires through the eyepiece of the telescope. Rotate the eyepiece until the cross-wires are at an angle of 45° to the vertical. Withdraw the eyepiece until the cross-wires are blurred. Push the eyepiece slowly in until the cross-wires are just in focus, accommodation being relaxed. The image is then at infinity.

(2) The telescope is focused on a distant object. The slit of the collimator is illuminated by a sodium source and is viewed directly by the telescope in the straight-through position. The collimator is adjusted until a sharp image of the collimator slit is obtained.

(3) The prism is now adjusted so that the refracting edge of the prism is parallel to the axis of rotation of the prism table.

(a) Place the prism on the prism table so that one face P is perpendicular to the lines parallel to the line joining adjusting screws 2 and 3 (see *Figure 91.1*). The prism table is then rotated so that light from the collimator falls on faces P and Q.

(b) Rotate the telescope until an image of the slit is seen by reflection from face P. Screws 2 and 3 are adjusted until the image is seen centrally in the field of the telescope. The telescope is then rotated until an image of the slit is seen by reflection from face Q. If the slit is not central in the field of view then only screw 1 is adjusted. Adjustment of this screw rotates face P in its own plane. Hence the previous adjustment will not be altered since reflections from face P will be undisturbed if face P is rotated in its own plane.

(c)   Rotate the telescope and check that the reflection from face P is still central. If not repeat steps (a) and (b) until the image of the slit is seen centrally by reflection from both faces P and Q.

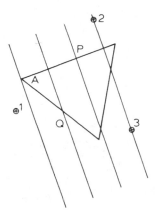

Figure 91.1. The prism is placed on the table so that face P is perpendicular to the lines parallel to the line joining adjusting screws 2 and 3. The prism table is rotated so that parallel light from the collimator slit falls on the prism faces P and Q. Rotate the telescope to receive an image of the collimator slit by reflection from face P. Adjust screws 2 and 3 until the image is central in the field of the telescope. Rotate the telescope to obtain an image from face Q. If the slit image is not central use only screw 1. This rotates face P in its own plane and hence will not affect the reflection from this face

Measurement of the refracting angle of the prism

(1)   *First method.* The prism is placed on the prism table so that light is reflected from both faces P and Q. The telescope is then rotated until the image is observed on the cross-wires. The telescope reading T_2 (see *Figure 91.2*) is determined. The reading T_1 for the other face is then obtained. The difference between these two readings $T_2 - T_1$ is 2A, where A is the refracting angle of the prism.

(2)   *Second method.* The prism is placed on the prism table and the image of the slit is seen by reflection from face Q. The telescope is then clamped. The reading of the prism table is obtained. The prism table is then rotated until an image of the slit is again observed; this will be by reflection from face P. The new position of the prism table is recorded. The difference between the two readings of the prism table is $180° - A$.

Figure 91.2. Measurement of the apical angle of the prism. The prism is placed on the prism table so that the refracting angle A faces the collimator. Light is reflected from both faces of the prism. Readings T_1 and T_2 of the telescope are obtained and the difference between these two readings is 2A

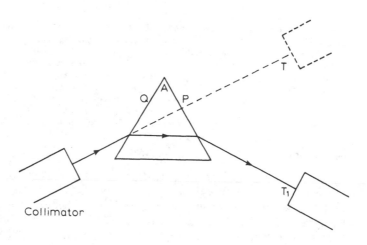

Figure 91.3. Measurement of angle of minimum deviation. At minimum deviation the path of light through a prism is symmetrical. The position T_1 of the telescope is observed and recorded. The prism is removed, and the straight-through position T of the telescope is determined. Then the angle of minimum deviation is $T - T_1$

332

Determination of refractive index by the position of minimum deviation

The prism is placed in a position near that of minimum deviation. The prism table and telescope are clamped and the slow motion adjustment of both prism table and telescope are used to determine the precise position of minimum deviation. This position is obtained when, with the telescope clamped, the prism table is rotated by means of the slow motion adjustment, and although the prism table is rotated in one direction the image of the slit advances to the intersection of the cross-wires seen in the telescope eyepiece but then recedes. The telescope is then in the position T_1 (see *Figure 91.3*). The position T_1 is recorded. The prism is removed and the straight-through position T is obtained. Then the angle of minimum deviation is $T - T_1$.

The prism is replaced on the prism table, and the table rotated so that the situation of *Figure 91.4* is obtained. The position of minimum

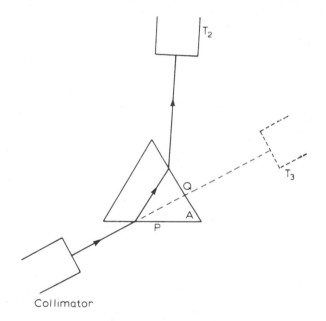

Collimator

Figure 91.4. Compare with Figure 91.3. The prism table is rotated so that parallel light from the collimator is incident first on face P and the path of light through the prism is symmetrical. Position T_2 of the telescope is determined. The prism is then removed and the straight-through position T_3 is obtained. Then the angle of minimum deviation is $T_2 - T_3$

deviation is again obtained as before and position T_2 of the telescope is determined. The prism is removed and the straight-through position T_3 of the telescope is determined. Then the angle of minimum deviation is $T_2 - T_3$.

The refractive index n of the prism is determined from

$$n = \frac{\sin \dfrac{A + D}{2}}{\sin \dfrac{A}{2}}$$

where A is the apical or refracting angle and D is the angle of minimum deviation.

Record your results as follows:

T	T_1	T_2	T_3	$T - T_1$ $= D_1$	$T_2 - T_3$ $= D_2$	$D =$ $\dfrac{D_1 + D_2}{2}$	A	$\sin \dfrac{A + D}{2}$	$\sin \dfrac{A}{2}$	$n =$	$\dfrac{\sin \dfrac{A + D}{2}}{\sin \dfrac{A}{2}}$

Experiment 92
LENS SYSTEM: PRINCIPAL PLANES AND EQUIVALENT LENS

Theory

If parallel light is incident on a lens system the image formed whether real or virtual could be equally well formed by a single lens of a certain power in a certain position. The power is the equivalent power of the system and the position is one of the principal planes of the system.

Consider *Figure 92.1*. This shows a lens system consisting of two thin lenses in air of focal powers F_1 and F_2 separated by a distance of d metres. After refraction by lenses F_1 and F_2 parallel light is focused at the point F'. It will be seen from the diagram that the same effect would be obtained if lenses F_1 and F_2 were replaced by a third lens of focal power F_3 placed in the position P' and of focal length $P'F'$. P' is called the second principal point. $P'F' = f'_e$ is called the second equivalent focal length. F' is called the second focal point of the lens system. The distance of F' from the second lens is called the back

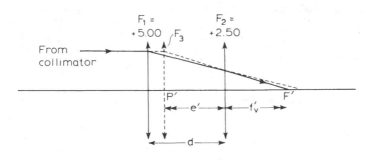

Figure 92.1

335

vertex focal length = f'_v, measured from the second lens to the second focal point.

The distance of the second principal point P' from the second lens, measured from the lens to P' is given the symbol e', and from the diagram

$$e' = f'_v - f'_e$$

Figure 92.2 shows the same lens system but parallel light is now incident on lens F_2, then on F_1 and is brought to a focus at the point F. It will be seen from the diagram that the same effect would be obtained if lenses F_1 and F_2 were replaced by a third lens of focal power F_3 placed in the position P and of focal length PF.

P is called the first principal point. PF = f_e is called the first equivalent focal length. F is called the first focal point of the lens system. The distance of F from the first lens is called the front vertex focal length = f_v, measured from the first lens to the first focal point.

PF and P'F' are of the same magnitude but are opposite in sign; hence $f'_e = -f_e$ for a lens system (just as a thin lens of focal power F_1 has first and second focal lengths f_1 and f'_1, where $f'_1 = -f_1$). The distance of the first principal point P from the first lens, measured from the first lens to P, is given the symbol e, and from the diagram, having regard to signs,

$$e = f_v - f_e$$

If f'_e and f_e are measured in metres the equivalent power F_e of the lens system is defined as

$$-\frac{1}{f_e} = \frac{1}{f'_e} = F_e$$

and it can be shown that

$$F_e = F_1 + F_2 - dF_1F_2$$

where d is measured in metres.

We define also:

The front vertex power $F_v = -\dfrac{1}{f_v}$

The back vertex power $F'_v = \dfrac{1}{f'_v}$

LENS SYSTEM: PRINCIPAL PLANES AND EQUIVALENT LENS

Figure 92.2

Apparatus

Optical bench, collimator, telescope, two thin lenses to form a lens system with an equivalent power equal to the power of the third lens provided, and a screen.

Procedure

(1)   Adjust the collimator to give parallel light. This is done by using the telescope which has previously been used to view a distant object or by the plane mirror method of Experiment 24.

(2)   The focal powers of the three lenses F_1, F_2 and F_3 are determined by auto-collimation. Four readings should be taken for each lens and the average of these readings is the focal power.

(3)   Use the two weaker lenses F_1 and F_2 to give a system with an equivalent power equal to the power of the third lens F_3 for a separation d metres.

As an example let $F_1 = + 5.00$ D
$$F_2 = + 2.50 \text{ D}$$
$$d = 10 \text{ cm } (0.1\text{m})$$
Then $F_3 = + 6.25$ D

(4)   Set up the components as shown in *Figure 92.3*.

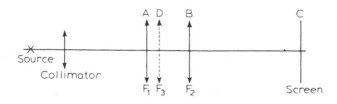

Figure 92.3

337

(a)   Light from the collimator is parallel; hence the screen will be at the second focal point of the lens system when a sharp image is formed on the screen. Record the positions of lens and screen.

(b)   Lenses F_1 and F_2 are removed, the screen is unaltered in position and lens F_3, the equivalent thin lens, is inserted. This is moved until a sharp image is obtained on the screen. Record the position of F_3.

(5)   Repeat for varying positions on the optical bench at least six times.

(6)   Record your results as shown below.

Positions				Distances		
Lens F_1	Lens F_2	Image	Lens F_3	Distance of lens F_3 from lens F_2 = BD	Back vertex focal length =BC	Equiv. focal length = DC
A	B	C	D	e'	f'_v	f'_e

(7)   The positions of F_1 and F_2 should be reversed and a similar determination of the first focal point F and first principal point P should be carried out.

(8)   Using the average of your readings, draw a full-scale diagram (if possible) to show the positions of the principal and focal points.

Verify that $e' = f'_v - f'_e$

$$e = f_v - f_e$$

and $f'_e = - f_e$

Experiment 93
EQUIVALENT FOCAL LENGTH:
NEWTON'S EQUATION

Theory

In Experiment 48 we derived Newton's equation $xx' = ff'$ for a thin lens. It can be shown that this is true for a lens system where f and f' are the first and second equivalent focal lengths respectively.

Apparatus

Optical bench, collimator, telescope, two thin lenses $+ 5.00$ D and $+ 2.50$ D, and a screen.

Procedure

(1) The two lenses are set up with a separation of 10 cm, approximately midway on the optical bench. By the method of Experiments 24, 25 or 48, the first and second focal points are determined. Their positions are recorded.

(2) The object is placed a distance x from the first focal point and the image of the object is found. The distance x' of the image from the second focal point is determined.

(3) Measure the size of the object h and of the corresponding image h'. The lateral magnification $m = h'/h$. Verify that

$$m = -\frac{x'}{f_e'} = -\frac{f_e}{x}$$

(4)　Vary the position of the object so that x changes by values of 1 cm and obtain the corresponding value x'.

Verify that for each set of observations

$$m = -\frac{x'}{f'_e} = -\frac{f_e}{x}$$

(5)　Record your results as shown below.

The record should show the positions of the optical components and from these x and x' can be determined. The values of x and x' should show that xx' is a constant and is equal to $-f'^2_e$.

(6)　Now $xx' = -f'^2_e$

or $x = -\dfrac{1}{x'} f'^2_e$

A graph of x against $1/x'$ will give a straight line whose gradient has the value $-f'^2_e$.

(7)　Calculate the equivalent power F_e from $F_e = F_1 + F_2 - dF_1 F_2$ and compare your results.

For guidance a set of results is given in *Figure 94.1*. From these:

$x = -17^1/_3$

$x' = 14.8$

$xx' = -256.5$

$f'_e = \sqrt{(256.5)}$

$\quad = 16.02$ cm

$m = -\dfrac{x'}{f'_e} = -0.924$

and $m = -\dfrac{f_e}{x} = -0.924$

Object	Position of F	Position of F'	Position of 1st lens	Position of 2nd lens	Position of image	x	x'	xx'	f'

Experiment 94
LENS SYSTEM, CONJUGATE FOCI

Theory

This experiment is designed to show that the application of the conjugate foci equation

$$L' = L + F$$

can be applied directly to a lens system, $L' = 1/l'$, $L = 1/l$, where:

l' is the distance of the image from the second principal plane, measured from the plane to the image.

l is the distance of the object from the first principal plane, measured from the plane to the object.

F is the equivalent power.

Apparatus

Optical bench; lens holders; object screen; + 8.00 D, + 10.00 D, − 8.00 D and − 10.00 D lenses.

Procedure

(1) A number of different lens systems are set up on the optical bench and the position of the principal planes calculated for each system.

The systems are:

	F_1	F_2	d, cm
(i)	+ 10.00 D	+ 8.00 D	6
(ii)	+ 10.00 D	− 8.00 D	6
(iii)	+ 8.00 D	+ 10.00 D	11
(iv)	− 8.00 D	− 10.00 D	8
(v)	+ 10.00 D	+ 10.00 D	15

341

(2)   The positions of the first and second principal planes can be conveniently marked on the optical bench with a pencil.

(3)   The image formed by the lens system is determined, and the distance l of the object is measured from the first principal plane, and the conjugate distance l' is measured from the second principal plane. This is repeated for different object distances. Note that for systems of negative focal power an auxiliary positive lens must be used to produce a real image.

(4)   Record your results as shown below for each lens system.

Calculation						Experiment			
F_1	F_2	d	F by calculation	e'	e	l	l'	F by conjugate foci

Compare the equivalent power determined by conjugate foci with the theoretical value obtained from the equation $F = F_1 + F_2 - dF_1F_2$.

(5) For guidance the calculations for the above systems are given on a separate page together with a model calculation to illustrate the method.

Calculation of the positions of the principal points, i.e. the distances e' and e

For two thin lenses in air of focal powers F_1, F_2, and of separation d it can be shown that $e' = \dfrac{-dF_1}{F}$ and $e = \dfrac{dF_2}{F}$

Then for the five lens systems we have:

(i) $F = 10 + 8 - \dfrac{6}{100} \times 10 \times 8$

$= + 13.2$ D

$e' = -6 \times 10/13.2$

$= -4.55$ cm

$e = 6 \times 8/13.2$

$= 3.64$ cm

(ii) $F = +10 - 8 - \dfrac{6}{100} \times 10 \times (-8)$

$$= + 2.48 \text{ D}$$
$$e' = - 6 \times 10/2.48$$
$$= - 24.19 \text{ cm}$$
$$e = 6 \times (- 8)/2.48$$
$$= - 19.35 \text{ cm}$$

(iii) $\quad F = + 8 + 10 - \dfrac{11}{100} \times 8 \times 10$

$$= + 9.20 \text{ D}$$
$$e' = - 11 \times 8/9.2$$
$$= - 9.56 \text{ cm}$$
$$e = 11 \times 10/9.2$$
$$= 11.96 \text{ cm}$$

(iv) $\quad F = - 8 - 10 - \dfrac{8}{100} \times (- 8) \times (- 10)$

$$= - 24.4 \text{ D}$$
$$e' = - 8 \times (- 8)/(24.4)$$
$$= - 2.62 \text{ cm}$$
$$e = 8 \times (- 10)/(- 24.4)$$
$$= 3.28 \text{ cm}$$

(v) $\quad F = + 10 + 10 - \dfrac{15}{100} \times 10 \times 10$

$$= + 5.00 \text{ D}$$
$$e' = - 15 \times 10/5$$
$$= - 75 \text{ cm}$$
$$e = 15 \times 10/5$$
$$= 75 \text{ cm}$$

Figure 94.1 shows the positions of the principal planes of a lens system with $F_1 = + 5.00$, $F_2 = + 2.50$, $d = 10$ cm. We will consider the formation of the image of an object $29^1/_3$ cm in front of the first lens, by the lens system, using the following methods:

Figure 94.1

(a) By conjugate foci applied to each lens in turn.
(b) By conjugate foci with reference to the principal planes.

(a) $l_1 = -29\frac{1}{3}$ cm; hence $L_1 = -3.409$ D

$$L'_1 = L_1 + F_1 = -3.409 \text{ D} + 5 \text{ D}$$
$$= +1.5909 \text{ D}$$
$$l'_1 = 62.857 \text{ cm}$$

This image acts as a virtual object for the second lens where

$$l_2 = 62.857 - 10$$
$$= 52.857 \text{ cm}$$
$$L'_2 = L_2 + F_2 = 1.8919 \text{ D} + 2.50 \text{ D}$$
$$= 4.3919 \text{ D}$$
$$l'_2 = 22.769 \text{ cm}$$

Hence the final image is 22.769 cm behind the second lens.

(b) By inspection of *Figure 93.1* it is seen that the object distance with regard to the first principal plane is $-33\frac{1}{3}$ cm.

Hence $L = -3.00$ D

$$L' = L + F, \text{ where F is the equivalent power}$$
$$L' = -3 \text{ D} + 6.25 \text{ D}$$
$$= +3.25 \text{ D}$$
$$l' = 30.769 \text{ cm}$$

Hence the final image is formed 30.769 cm behind the second principal plane. Since this plane is 8 cm in front of the second lens the final image is $30.769 - 8 = 22.769$ cm behind the second lens, which is exactly the same result as in method (a).

A third method is using Newton's equation, which has already been considered in Experiment 48.

Experiment 95
NEWTON'S RINGS

Description

Newton's Rings are observed if two polished surfaces of nearly equal curvature are placed in contact, and viewed either by reflection or transmission. They are interference fringes and can be seen to be coloured if white light is used, or light and dark and more extensive if a monochromatic light source is used.

Figure 95.1

345

Figure 95.1 indicates the way the apparatus is set up to view the rings by reflection. The rings originate from the thin film trapped between the two surfaces of nearly similar curvature. (The two plates may have been supplied clamped together.) If the experiment is repeated with water between the surfaces the rings will be fainter and closer together.

Theory

In *Figure 95.2* BAC is the trace of a spherical surface of large radius of curvature r, in contact at the point A of a flat optical surface. Since there is circular symmetry the rings are concentric circles. Let the film enclosed between the two surfaces have refractive index n. If there is perfect optical contact there is a central dark circular patch. The dark ring surrounding this central spot is the first ring (k = 1), and the dark rings are counted outwards from this position.

Let t be the thickness of the film for a particular ring number k, radius y. Then it can be shown that for normal incidence

$$t = \frac{k\lambda}{2n} \qquad \ldots \ (1)$$

where λ is the wavelength of the light illuminating the surfaces.

From *Figure 95.2* it is seen that the sag s of surface trace BAC is of the same magnitude as t.

Since the surface has a large radius of curvature (focal power 0.12 D say) then the approximate sag formula can be used.

Hence
$$s = \frac{y^2}{2r}$$

where r is the radius of curvature of the surface.

From equations (1) and (2)
$$\frac{k\lambda}{2n} = \frac{y^2}{2r}$$

Rearranging
$$y^2 = \frac{k\lambda r}{n}$$

Thus if y^2 is plotted against k a straight line of gradient $\lambda r/n$ is obtained.

If λ and n are known, r can be calculated. If λ and r are known, n can be calculated.

Procedure

(1)   Adjust the travelling microscope so that the cross-wires intersect the central spot of the circular pattern (k = 0 for central dark patch).

(2)   Move the microscope to the left until the cross-wires intersect the fifth dark ring (k = 5).
Record this position.

(3)   Repeat for the rings where k = 10, 15, 20, 25.

(4)   Move the microscope to the right until the cross-wires intersect the central spot.

(5)   Move the microscope to the left and record the readings for the rings where k = 5, 10, 15, 20, 25.

(6)   Record your results as shown below.

k = Ring number	Microscope reading		Ring diameter	Ring radius = y	y^2
	Left	Right			
5					
10					
15					
20					
25					

(7)   Plot a graph of y^2 against ring number k. The gradient of the slope will be λr for an air film since n = 1. Since λ is known r can be calculated.

(8)   Repeat the experiment with water between the surfaces. It will be found that the rings will be fainter and closer together. The gradient of the slope will be $\lambda r/n$ where n is the refractive index of water. Since λ and r are known, n can be calculated.

Note. – The straight line of the graphs will go through the origin only if there is perfect optical contact at A. This perfect optical contact does not always happen.

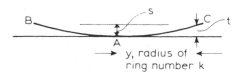

Figure 95.2. BAC is the trace of a spherical surface of large radius of curvature in optical contact at A with a flat surface. If there is perfect contact there is a dark spot at A

347

Experiment 96
FRONT CENTRAL OPTIC RADIUS OF A CONTACT LENS

Theory

When the physical fit of a contact lens has been determined, the back central optic radius r_2 is fixed. The back vertex power F'_v is known; hence if a central thickness of the contact lens is given, the front central optic radius can be calculated. This information is usually given to the contact lens manufacturer by the practitioner, who relies on the manufacturer to calculate r_1 the front central optic radius.

Since the back vertex power of the contact lens is F'_v, then the vergence of the wavefront at the second surface, power F_2, is

$$F'_v - F_2 \qquad \dots \text{(1)}$$

The reciprocal of this vergence is

$$f'_1 - \frac{t}{n} \qquad \dots \text{(2)}$$

See *Figure 96.1.*

Figure 96.1. F'_v is the back vertex power of a spectacle lens, physical thickness t, surface powers F_1 and F_2

Hence if f'_1 and t are expressed in mm, then from equations (1) and (2)

$$\frac{1000}{F'_v - F_2} = f'_1 - \frac{t}{n} \qquad \ldots \text{(3)}$$

If r_1 is expressed in mm then

$$f'_1 = \frac{r_1}{n - 1} \qquad \ldots \text{(4)}$$

From equations (3) and (4)

$$r_1 = (n - 1)\left(\frac{1000}{F'_v - F_2} + \frac{t}{n}\right) \qquad \ldots \text{(5)}$$

Apparatus

Radiuscope, dial gauge, contact lens of known back vertex power, focimeter.

Procedure

(1)   Record the number of the contact lens.

(2)   Verify, with the focimeter, that the back vertex power of the contact lens is correct.

(3)   Determine the back central optic radius (BCOR) r_2 using the radiuscope.

(4)   Determine the central thickness t.

(5)   Determine the front central optic radius (FCOR) using equaation (5). Assume the refractive index is 1.49.

(6)   Record your results as follows.

Lens No.	BCOR r_2	t	F'_v	FCOR r_1 by calculation

Comment on what accuracy is required for r_1 and r_2 so that F'_v is correct to ± 0.25 D.

Experiment 97
NEAR VISION EFFECTIVITY ERROR

Theory

It has been pointed out in several earlier experiments that spectacle lenses are numbered in terms of their back vertex powers. The back vertex power of a lens expresses the vergence in the refracted pencil as it leaves the back surface of the lens when the vergence in the pencil incident upon the front surface is zero. The light is assumed to originate from a distant object.

In the case of a distant object we can say that the back vertex power represents the change in vergence which is produced by a spectacle lens upon the incident light, that is, the vergence which is impressed by the lens. This follows from the conjugate foci relationship, $L' = L + F$, since, when $L_1 = 0$, we can write:

$$L'_2 = F'_v$$

When a spectacle lens is used for near vision, however, we no longer have a distant object and back vertex power notation provides only an approximate indication of the vergence impressed by a lens.

In the case of a near object, the vergence which leaves the back surface of the lens, L'_2, is given by the somewhat lengthy paraxial expression:-

$$L'_2 = \frac{L_1 + F_1 + F_2 - (t/n)F_2(L_1 + F_1)}{1 - (t/n)\,(L_1 + F_1)}$$

where L_1 is the incident vergence from the near object, F_1 and F_2 are the individual surface powers, t represents the axial thickness and n the refractive index of the lens. It should be noted that, in the case of a distant object, L_1 is zero and the expression reduces to the back vertex power relationship given in Experiment 51.

Alternatively, L'_2 can be found from a paraxial ray-trace through the lens.

350

It will be realised that L'_2 cannot be found simply by adding the incident vergence, L_1 to the back vertex power of the lens. A correction factor needs to be taken into account. This correction factor is called the near vision effectivity error, **NVEE.**

There are several instances where difficulties may arise when prescribing lenses for near vision which result from a strict adherence to vertex power notation.

The most important one is the problem of different near vision effectivity errors between the trial lens used during refraction and the final lens which the subject is dispensed.

$$L'_2 = L_1 + F'_v + NVEE$$

Figure 97.1 The problem of Near Vision Effectivity Error.

A typical case is illustrated in Figure 97.1 which compares the performance in near vision of a +10.00 D trial lens of the form most commonly employed in the UK, a reduced aperture design where the curved surface is intended to face the eye, with that of a final lens of the same back vertex power.

For a near object at −33.3 cm the vergence arriving at the front surface of each lens is −3.00 D. Assigning suitable curves and thicknesses to each lens we find, by paraxial ray-tracing, that the vergence leaving the back surface of the trial lens in near vision is +7.02 D whereas the vergence leaving the back surface of the final lens is only +6.58 D.

351

Near vision effectivity error, NVEE, is defined as the difference between the value, L'_2, which is the actual vergence leaving the back surface of the lens, and the anticipated vergence, $L_1 + F'_v$, which is the sum of the incident vergence, (L_1), and the back vertex power of the lens, (F'_v), i.e. $L'_2 = L_1 + F'_v + NVEE$.

The NVEE can be looked upon as a correction factor which must be taken into account when the form of the lens is changed in the case of lenses which are prescribed for near vision.

For the example in hand, the NVEE of the trial lens is, the very small value, $+0.02$ D, but for the final lens it is -0.42 D.

If a difference of this magnitude is ignored, say in cases of aphakia where the subject has no extra accommodation in order to compensate for the loss in power, the final lenses may well be useless to the wearer. It is for this reason that it has been suggested that, in cases of aphakia, the reading addition should be increased by $+0.50$ or $+0.75$ in order to replace the loss in plus power which occurs when the form is changed from that of the trial lens to that of the final lens.

NVEE depends upon the position of the near object and the form and thickness of the lens. For a given object distance the error increases as the lens becomes more steeply curved, or, as the thickness increases.

In the case of minus lenses and low-power plus lenses the errors due to near vision effectivity are negligible. However, for moderate and high-power plus lenses the errors cannot be ignored.

Typical near vision effectivity errors are given in the accompanying table for a series of modern plus lenses which are assumed to be used for near vision at -33.3 cm and -40.0 cm.

BVP	NVEE	
	-33.3 cm	-40.0 cm
$+3.00$	-0.12 D	-0.10 D
$+6.00$	-0.20 D	-0.18 D
$+9.00$	-0.38 D	-0.33 D
$+12.00$	-0.46 D	-0.39 D
$+15.00$	-0.57 D	-0.49 D

In practice, these values can be measured by the focimeter when an auxiliary lens is employed as described in Experiment 98.

In this experiment it is shown how to calculate the error, and how to specify the powers of lenses required for near vision which exhibit equal errors of near vision effectivity.

Procedure

(1) Accurately transpose the lens, if necessary, so that both surface powers are known.

(2) Using the conjugate foci relationship (or the expression given above) trace a ray of light from the near point through each surface of the lens to determine the vergence, L'_2, leaving the back surface in near vision.

The ray-tracing sequence is as follows (distances assumed to be given in mm):

$$L_1 = 1000/l_1$$
$$L'_1 = L_1 + F_1$$
$$l'_1 = 1000/L'_1$$
$$l_2 = l'_1 - t/n$$
$$L_2 = 1000/l_2$$
$$L'_2 = L_2 + F_2$$

(3) Compare the vergence leaving the back surface, L'_2, found in step 2, with the value obtained by adding L_1 and F'_v. The NVEE is the difference

$$L'_2 - (L_1 + F'_v).$$

If the lens for which the NVEE has been found in the sequence above is a trial lens it is possible to calculate the specification of a final lens which will have the same effect as the trial lens as follows.

(4) Using the conjugate foci relationship, trace a ray back through the lens starting, this time, with the value of L'_2 obtained in step 2, in order to determine the power of the front surface which would give the same value of L'_2 for the given object distance, L_1.

The ray-tracing sequence for this reverse trace is as follows:

$$L_2 = L'_2 - F_2$$
$$l_2 = 1000/L_2$$
$$l'_1 = l_2 + t/n$$
$$L'_1 = 1000/l'_1$$
$$F_1 = L'_1 - L_1$$

(5) Now that the individual surface powers of the near vision lens are known we can find its back vertex power using the method outlined in Experiment 51.

Examples

(1) A $+10.00$ D lens intended for use in near vision at one-third metre from the front surface of the lens, is made in glass of refractive index 1.5 with a -3.00 base curve and an axial thickness of 9 mm. Find the near vision effectivity error.

The nominal front curve of the lens is $+13.00$ D and the compensated front curve, using the methods outlined in Experiment 64, is $+12.06$ D. By means of the ray-tracing procedure outlined above:

$$
\begin{aligned}
l_1 &= -333.3 \text{ mm} \\
L_1 &= -3.00 \text{ D} \\
L'_1 &= +9.06 \text{ D} \\
l'_1 &= +110.38 \text{ mm} \\
l_2 &= +104.38 \text{ mm} \\
L_2 &= +9.58 \\
L'_2 &= +6.58 \text{D} \quad \text{(see Figure 97.1)}
\end{aligned}
$$

The anticipated vergence leaving the lens is $L_1 + F'_v$ which is $+7.00$ D.

The NVEE is -0.42 D.

(2) An eye is corrected for near vision at 35 cm from the cornea, by a $+14.00$ D trial lens made with a plane front surface and an axial thickness of 4 mm, the vertex distance of the trial lens being 12 mm. The final lens which the subject is to wear is to be made with a -3.00 D back curve, an axial thickness of 10.0 mm and mounted at the same vertex distance. Find the back vertex power of the lens which must be ordered. (Assume n = 1.523 for each lens).

The back surface of the trial lens is $+14.00$ D and the near point lies 334 mm from its front surface. The vergence leaving the back surface of the trial lens in near vision can be found from the ray-tracing sequence outlined above.

$$
\begin{aligned}
l_1 &= -334 \text{ mm} \\
L_1 &= -2.99 \text{ D} \\
L'_1 &= -2.99 \text{ D} \\
l'_1 &= -334 \text{ mm} \\
l_2 &= -336.63 \text{ mm} \\
L_2 &= -2.97 \text{ D} \\
L'_2 &= +11.03 \text{ D}
\end{aligned}
$$

In order to determine the back vertex power of the final lens we must find the front surface power which will produce the same value for L'_2

when the object distance measured to the front surface of the final lens is -328 mm.

Hence
$$L'_2 = +11.03 \text{ D}$$
$$L_2 = +14.03 \text{ D}$$
$$l_2 = +71.28 \text{ mm}$$
$$l'_1 = +77.84 \text{ mm}$$
$$L'_1 = +12.85 \text{ D}$$
$$F_1 = +15.90 \text{ D}.$$

Now that we know the front surface power for the final lens we can find its back vertex power. Using the method given in Experiment 51 we find:

$$F'_v = +14.75 \text{ D}.$$

Prescriptions

The following lenses are intended for near vision use at 35 cm from the front surface. Assuming that they are made from glass of refractive index 1.523 find the NVEE in each case.

(1) $+8.00$ D, with back curve -4.00 D and $t = 6.0$ mm
(2) $+5.00$ D, with back curve -6.00 D and $t = 5.0$ mm
(3) $+12.00$ D, with back curve $+12.00$ D and $t = 9.0$ mm
(4) $+12.00$ D, with back curve $+5.90$ D and $t = 9.0$ mm
(5) $+12.00$ D, with back curve -4.00 D and $t = 9.0$ mm

(6)   What back vertex power would need to be ordered for the lens described in Q.(5) if it is required to have the same effect in near vision as the trial lens described in:-

(i)   Question (3)?
(ii)   Question (4)?

Experiment 98
MEASUREMENT OF SPECTACLE LENSES FOR NEAR VISION

Theory

The focimeter is a vertex power measuring instrument designed to measure the vertex power of a spectacle lens. When the lens is placed in the focimeter with its back surface in contact with the lens rest or stop, the instrument records the **back** vertex power of the lens. This is the value which we usually require to confirm since spectacle lenses are numbered in terms of their back vertex powers.

Back vertex power notation is used because a spectacle lens corrects an eye for distance vision when its second principal focus, F', coincides with the eye's far point, M_R (Figure 98.1). The purpose of the correcting lens, for distance vision, is to produce an image of a distant object at the eye's far point. Since the far point is conjugate with the macula, the eye's own optical system produces a final image, in sharp focus, at the macula.

Figure 91.1 The spectacle lens in distance vision

When we determine the back vertex power of a lens by means of the focimeter, the instrument's power control knob is used to adjust the position of the target, T, until its image, T', lies at the second principal focus of the lens (Figure 98.2). Parallel light then emerges from the front surface of the lens under test and a sharp image of the target is seen through the focimeter's viewing system, usually a telescope, when in correct adjustment for infinity.

Figure 98.2 Vertex power measurement by the focimeter.

Comparison of figures 98.1 and 98.2 demonstrates that the focimeter exactly simulates the method by which a spectacle lens corrects an eye for distance vision. The ray paths are identical.

Occasionally, we also need to measure the front vertex power of a spectacle lens, typically to confirm the reading addition of a bifocal or multifocal lens when the segment is situated on the front surface of the lens.

Front vertex power is measured simply by reversing the lens in the instrument in order to place the front surface of the lens in contact with the stop. It is necessary to adopt this procedure when measuring the reading addition of a bifocal which has a front-surface segment since the manufacturer of the bifocal surface has to predetermine the addition at the semi-finished stage of lens manufacture. He cannot know the final thickness of the finished lens and, hence, cannot incorporate any compensation for thickness at the bifocal surface production stage.

However, neither front vertex power measurement nor back vertex power measurement give a full account of how a spectacle lens performs in near vision.

Back vertex power is a measure of the vergence leaving the back surface of a lens when the incident vergence on the front vertex is zero. The light is assumed to originate from a distant object.

In near vision we are not dealing with a distant object and the back vertex system of numbering spectacle lenses only provides an approximate indication of the vergence impressed by a lens in near vision.

In order to measure the vergence leaving a spectacle lens under near vision conditions we must employ an auxiliary lens which is placed in contact with the front surface of the lens under test and is designed to simulate the ray-path in near vision.

For near vision at −33.3 cm we would use a −3.00 auxiliary lens. For near vision at −40.0 cm we would use a −2.50 D auxiliary lens and so on. A trial lens is ideal for the purpose. Strictly the auxiliary lens should be plano-concave in form and placed with the curved surface in contact with the front surface of the lens under test. However, since the auxiliary lens is of low power and likely to be thin, its form, from a practical point of view, is really immaterial.

357

The optical principle is explained in Figures 98.3 and 98.4 which confirm that the action of the auxiliary lens is to enable the focimeter to simulate the ray-path in near vision.

The spectacle lens in near vision

Figure 98.3 The spectacle lens in near vision

Measurement of L'₂ by the focimeter

Figure 98.4 Measurement of spectacle lenses in NV.

The action of the −3.00 D auxiliary lens shown in the figure is, effectively, to reduce the front surface power by −3.00 D which has exactly the same mathematical effect as an incident vergence of −3.00 D upon the front surface.

Needless to say, if we wish to duplicate the effect of a lens for near vision we should not match its back vertex power but, rather, the vergence which the lens impresses in near vision. In other words, two lenses of different forms will have the same effect in near vision if the vergence leaving the back surface of each lens is the same when measured by the focimeter with an auxiliary lens in contact with the front surface of the lens under test.

Thus, the focimeter can be used to measure near vision effectivity errors and to give a full account of the performance of a lens in near vision.

Apparatus

Focimeter; auxiliary lenses of powers -2.50 and -3.00; plus lenses of moderate to high power (say $+4.00$ and above) to test.

Procedure

(1) Measure the back vertex power of the lens under test by means of the focimeter.

(2) Place the auxiliary minus lens in contact with the front surface of the lens under test and read the "power" of the combination by means of the focimeter. The reading obtained is the vergence leaving the back surface of the lens, L'_2, when the incident vergence is the same as the power of the auxiliary lens.

(3) Obtain the anticipated value for L'_2 by adding the power of the auxiliary lens to the back vertex power of the lens.

(4) Determine the near vision effectivity error by subtracting the anticipated value obtained in step 3 from the measured value obtained in step 2.

Record your results as follows.

Auxiliary lens	F'v of lens under test	Measured value of L'_2	$L_1 + F'_v$	NVEE
-3.00	$+10.00$	$+6.50$	$+7.00$	-0.50
-2.50	$+6.00$	$+3.25$	$+3.50$	-0.25

Experiment 99
MEASUREMENT OF THE MECHANICAL ADDITION OF BIFOCAL LENSES

Theory

The reading addition of a bifocal or multifocal lens is defined as the difference between the vertex powers of the reading and distance portions measured from the surface which incorporates the segment. Hence, in the case of front-surface segment designs, the addition is the difference between the front vertex powers of the reading and distance portions. This method of measurement often gives rise to difficulties especially in the case of bifocal lenses where the distance portion is positive.

The problem is illustrated in Figure 99.1 which shows the readings which would be obtained when the prescription +4.00 Add +2.00 is checked by means of the focimeter. If the lens has been correctly made then the back vertex power of the distance portion should read +4.00 D.

+4·00   Add 2·00

+4·00

A   +3·82   B   +5·82

Add = B − A = +2·00

Figure 99.1 Measurement of the reading addition

The addition which is provided by the manufacturer is the difference between the **front** vertex powers of the reading and distance portions. These are measured with the spectacles reversed in the instrument. If the lens has been correctly made then this difference should be +2.00 D.

If we were to measure the difference between the **back** vertex powers of the distance and reading portions the readings would indicate that the addition is greater than the prescribed value (Figure 99.2)

+4·00   Add 2·00

+6·25?

Add = 2·25?

Figure 99.2 Measurement of the "over-plus" syndrome.

In this case we might deduce that the reading addition measured from the back of the lens, and that which the patient is actually being given, is +2.25 D!

A better indication of the real effect of the segment in near vision is obtained by measuring the **mechanical addition** of the lens which can be defined as the difference between the vergences leaving the reading and distance portions when the vergence incident upon the front surface is that which arrives from the near point.

Clearly, the mechanical addition, which can be measured with the assistance of an auxiliary lens as described in Experiment 98, represents the real difference between the vergences leaving the reading and distance portions in near vision. In other words, it indicates the effect which is obtained when the wearer uses the segment compared with the effect which would be obtained if the segment was not there, i.e. the effect of a single vision lens whose power is equal to that of the distance portion.

The mechanical addition is measured by reading the vergences leaving the back surface of the lens through the distance and reading portions with an auxiliary lens in contact with the front surface. It is not necessary to reverse the lens in the instrument.

Typical values, which have been obtained from the lenses described below, will be discussed.

i) Glass solid bifocal - segment on back surface, axial thickness - t = 4.0 mm back surface = −6.00 D

		DP	RP	RP-DP
measured	BVP	+4.75	+7.50	+2.75
measured	L'_2	+1.62	+4.37	+2.75

ii) fused bifocal - segment on front surface

t = 3.8 mm   back surface = −5.00 D

		DP	RP	RP-DP
measured	BVP	+4.00	+6.62	+2.62
measured	FVP	+3.87	+6.37	+2.50
measured	L'_2	+0.87	+3.37	+2.50

iii) CR 39 lentic bifocal - segment on front surface
t = 9.7 mm   back surface = −2.25

		DP	RP	RP-DP
measured	BVP	+16.00	+19.75	+3.75
measured	FVP	+14.00	+17.00	+3.00
measured	L'_2	+12.37	+15.87	+3.50

Considering these examples individually, we see that in case (i), where the segment is situated on the concave surface of the lens, the measured addition is the same with or without the auxiliary lens. This is to be expected since the NVEE (−0.12 D) is the same for both the distance and the reading portions of the lens.

In case (ii), where the segment is situated on the convex surface of the lens and the axial thickness is not too great, the mechanical addition is the same, to within the accuracy of measurement, as the measured difference between the front vertex powers of the lens.

In case (iii), however, where the axial thickness of the lens is significant, the mechanical addition is greater than the measured difference between the front vertex powers. In order to avoid this over-plus syndrome, which is a well-known source of difficulty in practice, we should apply a correction factor to the prescribed reading addition in those cases where a bifocal design is dispensed with the segment on the front surface.

A suitable correction is given, for both crown glass, and for CR 39 material, by:-

$$-t.A_B.F_1/750$$

where t is the axial thickness of the lens in mm

A_B is the required reading addition

F_1 is the front surface power of the lens.

Since reading additions are normally manufactured in $+0.25$ D steps a suitable expression for the correction factor is:-

$$-INT (4 \times t \times A_B \times F_1/750 + 0.5)/4$$

which, of course, may easily be incorporated into a surfacing instruction program for the lens manufacturer.

Correction factors for the two examples quoted above, calculated from this latter expression would be:-

example ii) assuming F_1 = $+8.75$ correction = 0
example iii) assuming F_1 = $+16.32$ correction = -0.75

The purpose of this experiment is to measure the mechanical addition of bifocal lenses which have their segments on the front surface, and to compare the mechanical addition with the reading addition determined from the difference between the front vertex powers of each portion of the lens.

Apparatus

Focimeter; auxiliary lenses of powers -2.50 and -3.00; front-surface segment bifocal lenses to test; thickness calipers; lens measure.

Procedure

(1) Measure the back vertex power of the distance portion of the bifocal lens to determine the distance prescription of the lens.

(2) Measure the front vertex powers of the distance and reading portions of the lens. The difference between these represents the reading addition which has been provided by the manufacturer. (In the case of a solid bifocal, the manufacturer's addition can also be obtained with a lens measure since it will be the difference between the DP and the RP curves).

(3)   With the auxiliary lens held in contact with the front surface of the bifocal lens under test, place the back surface of the lens against the focimeter stop and read the "powers" of the distance and reading portions. These represent the L'_2 values for each portion as would be obtained by the wearer if he was viewing a near object through each portion. The difference between these two values is the mechanical addition of the lens.

(4)   If the mechanical addition which is found in step (3) is at least 0.12 D greater than the manufacturer's addition obtained in step (2), apply the expression for the correction factor in order to determine which addition would need to be ordered to provide a mechanical addition which matches the prescribed reading addition. (Use the thickness calipers and lens measure to obtain t and F_1).

Record your results as follows

	DP	RP	RP-DP (Add)	Correction factor
measured BVP	+8.00	+10.25	+2.25	−
measured FVP	+7.75	+9.75	+2.00	−
measured L'_2	+4.75	+7.00	+2.25	−0.25*

*F_1 and t found to be +10.50 and 6.0 mm respectively.

Experiment 100
MEASUREMENT OF THE REFRACTIVE INDEX
OF A SPECTACLE LENS

Theory

Spectacle lens materials are classified in terms of refractive index, n, as follows:

Normal Index	$n \geq 1.48$ but < 1.54
Mid index	$n \geq 1.54$ but < 1.64
High index	$n \geq 1.64$ but < 1.74
Very high index	$n \geq 1.74$.

The popularity of fashion spectacle frames with large eyesizes has led to an increase in the use of higher refractive index materials since this results in the finished lenses being thinner and lighter than when made in normal index materials. In practice, it may be necessary to determine the refractive index of an unknown lens. Several experiments given earlier in this book describe laboratory methods for the determination of refractive index but these often require the use of equipment which is unlikely to found in an optician's practice.

If the power of a spectacle lens is known then a good estimation of the refractive index of the lens can be obtained with the aid of a lens measure. The power of an unknown lens can be read in a focimeter and the surface curvatures obtained with the lens measure. If the thickness of the lens is ignored, then the refractive index of the lens material can be deduced from the ratio of the focimeter reading to the lens measure reading by means of the surface power relationship. Fortunately, in practice, higher index materials are usually employed for minus lenses since there is a noticeable reduction in edge thickness. Although plus lenses would also be thinner, the reduction in centre thickness is not so apparent to the observer.

A lens measure calibrated for a refractive index, n_{LM}, reads $(n_{LM} - 1)R$ when placed on a lens surface, whether the refractive index of the lens material is the same as that for which the lens measure is calibrated or not. R is the curvature of the surface, or if the thickness of the lens is ignored, R can be taken as the total curvature of the lens, $(R_1 - R_2)$. The true power of the lens, F_T, is $(n_T - 1)R$, where n_T is the true refractive index of the lens material. Since the curvature is constant in these two expressions it follows that:

$$F_T/(n_T - 1) = F_{LM}/(n_{LM} - 1).$$

F_T is the true power of the lens which can be obtained, for example, from the focimeter and F_{LM} is the sum of the two surface powers obtained with the lens measure.

n_T can then be determined from: $\quad n_T = 1 + (n_{LM} - 1)F_T/F_{LM}.$

Apparatus

Selection of lenses of different refractive indices; focimeter (or neutralizing set); lens measure.

Procedure

(1) Determine the power of the lens by means of the focimeter or by neutralization, F_T.

(2) Note the refractive index for which the lens measure has been scaled, n_{LM}. (It would normally be either 1.523 or 1.530 but some modern instruments have been calibrated for a plastics material of refractive index 1.500).

(3) Measure the surface powers of the lens with the lens measure and add these together to obtain the power of the lens according to the lens measure, F_{LM}.

(4) Find the refractive index of the lens from: $n_T = 1 + (n_{LM} - 1)F_T/F_{LM}$.

Record your results as follows.

Lens No.	Lens power F_T	Readings by lens measure F_1 F_2	Thin lens power $F_{LM} = (F_1 + F_2)$	n_T

Example

A lens measure calibrated for glass of refractive index 1.523 reads +4.00 and -10.00 when placed on a spectacle lens whose true power determined by focimeter is -8.00. What is the refractive index of the lens?

The thin lens power, F_{LM} (= $F_1 + F_2$) is -6.00, F_T is -8.00 and n_{LM} is 1.523.

Using $n_T = 1 + (n_{LM} - 1)F_T/F_{LM}$, $n_T = 1 + 0.523 \times 8/6 = 1.70$.

Note: Owing to the uncertainty of the individual readings you should not expect any accuracy better than two places of decimals from this experiment.

Experiment 101
MEASUREMENT OF THE ASPHERICITY
OF A CONICOIDAL SURFACE

Theory

Many spectacle lenses are made in aspheric form where the convex surface is (or closely resembles) a conicoid. A conicoidal surface is obtained upon rotation of a conic section around its major axis. The equation to a conic section can be written in the form:

$$y^2 = 2r_0x - px^2$$

where r_0 is the radius of curvature of the section at the vertex, or origin of the curve, x represents the sag of the curve at the diameter, 2y, and p defines the asphericity of the curve. The whole family of conic sections is illustrated in *Figure 101.1* and the name chosen to describe the curve depends upon the value of p.

When p > 1, the section is described as an oblate ellipse
p = 1, the section is a circle
0 < p < 1, the section is described as a prolate ellipse
p = 0, the section is a parabola
p < 0, the section is a hyperola.

Rotation of these conic sections around the x axis produces the conicoids, called respectively, oblate ellipsoids, the sphere, prolate ellipsoids, the paraboloid and the hyperboloid. Most aspheric lens series employ either a convex prolate ellipsoid or a convex hyperboloid for their front surfaces.

The sag of a conicoid, x, for a given chord diameter, 2y, may be found from:

$$x = y^2/\{r_0 + \sqrt{(r_0^2 - py^2)}\}.$$

It should be noted that when 1 is substituted for p, this expression gives the sag of a spherical surface.

For a prolate ellipsoidal surface whose vertex radius is 50mm and whose asphericity is defined as p = 0.40, the sag of the surface, x, at 60mm diameter may be found as follows:

Given: $r_0 = 50$, y = 30, p = +0.40,

$$x = y^2/\{r_0 + \sqrt{(r_0^2 - py^2)}\}$$

$$= 30^2/\{50 + \sqrt{(50^2 - 0.4 \times 30^2)}\}$$

$$= 9.35mm.$$

In the case of a hyperboloidal surface, where the value of p is negative, care should be taken to substitute the correct sign into the denominator of this sag equation.

For example, with a hyperboloidal surface whose vertex radius is 90mm and whose asphericity is defined as p = -1.50, the calculation for the sag of the surface at 70mm diameter is as follows.

Given: $r_0 = 90$, $y = 35$, $p = -1.50$,

$$x = y^2/\{r_0 + \sqrt{(r_0^2 - py^2)}\}$$

$$= 35^2/\{90 + \sqrt{(90^2 + 1.5 \times 35^2)}\}$$

$$= 6.46\text{mm}.$$

When the radius of curvature of the surface at the vertex, r_0, is known (or the true surface power of the curve at the vertex, F_0, and the refractive index of the lens material, n, are given, *nb.*, $r_0 = 1000(n - 1)/F_0$, as usual), then the p-value of the surface can be found by measuring the sag of the curve at two different diameters, i.e., by using two sagometers which have different chord values. In the workshop, sag gauges which have measuring diameters of 34mm, 40mm or 50mm may be found. Ideally, the greatest available difference, *eg*, the 34mm and 50mm gauges should be chosen.

If the sags, x_1 and x_2 of a conicoidal surface are known for two different semi-chord values, y_1 and y_2, then since the vertex radius is constant, from the equation for the conic section, $r_0 = (y^2 + px^2)/2x$,

$$(y_1^2 + px_1^2)/2x_1 = (y_2^2 + px_2^2)/2x_2^2$$

from which: $p = \dfrac{x_2 y_1^2 - x_1 y_2^2}{x_1 x_2 (x_2 - x_1)}$

Note: The sag gauge must be capable of measurement to the nearest 0.01mm. This should enable p to be given to one place of decimals from this experiment. To improve accuracy, the sags would need to be measured to three places of decimals! In order to check that the asphericity obtained from the experiment is reasonably close to its true value, it is recommended that the p-value should be substituted back into the sag equation given above to confirm that the sags obtained from the formula match those found with the sagometers.

Apparatus

Selection of aspheric lenses; two sag gauges with different bell diameters; calculator.

Procedure

(1) Measure the sag of the surface with the smaller diameter gauge. Record the result as x_1 and note (or measure, if not given) the semi-diameter of the smaller gauge, y_1.

(2) Measure the sag of the surface with the larger diameter gauge. Record the result as x_2 and note (or measure, if not given) the semi-diameter of the larger gauge, y_2.

(3) Use the relationship given above to calculate the value of p.

(4) In order to check that the asphericity which has been calculated in step 3 is reasonably accurate, substitute the p-value into the sag relationship for a conicoidal surface to ensure that the results agree with those read by the sag gauge.

Example

A lens made in a plastics material of refractive index 1.50 has a convex conicoidal surface of power +5.00D. The sags of this surface, measured with a 32mm sag gauge and a 50mm sag gauge are found to be 1.28mm and 3.14mm respectively. What is the p-value for the surface?

Given: $x_1 = 1.28$ when $y_1 = 16$ and $x_2 = 3.14$ when $y_2 = 25$.

$$\text{Since } p = \frac{x_2 y_1^2 - x_1 y_2^2}{x_1 x_2 (x_2 - x_1)}$$

$$\text{substituting the values, } p = \frac{3.14 \times 16^2 - 1.28 \times 25^2}{1.28 \times 3.14(3.14 - 1.28)}$$

$$= +0.5.$$

In order to check this value of p, it can be substituted back into the equation for the sag of a conicoid, $x - y^2/\{r_0 + \sqrt{(r_0^2 - py^2)}\}$.

The radius at the vertex is found from $r_0 = 1000(n - 1)/F_0 = 500/5 = 100$mm.

When $2y = 32$, $y = 16$ and $x = y^2/\{r_0 + \sqrt{(r_0^2 - py^2)}\}$

$$= 16^2/\{100 + \sqrt{(100^2 - 0.5 \times 16^2)}\}$$

$$= 1.28\text{mm}.$$

When $2y = 50$, $y = 25$ and $x = 25^2/\{100 + \sqrt{(100^2 - 0.5 \times 25^2)}\}$

$$= 3.15\text{mm}$$

which is sufficiently close to the measured value to assume that p does lie in the region of +0.5.

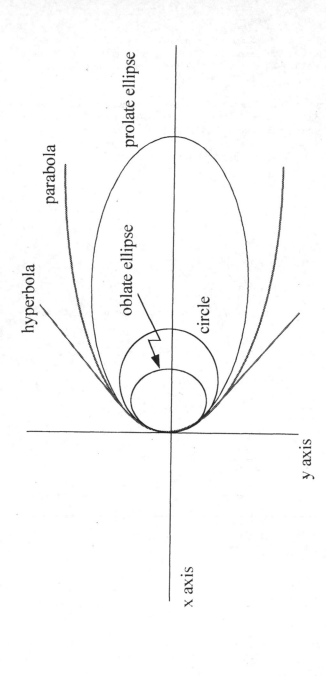

Figure 101.1 The conic sections $y^2 = 2r_o x - p x^2$

Appendix 1

STUDENTS' INSTRUCTION FORMS

TEST 1

Time allowed

Thirty minutes.

Lens set

Neutralizing set.

Instructions

You are required to record the identification number, prescription and form of any ten spherical lenses selected from the accompanying box.

Record your results as follows.

Name.............. Group............. Date..............
Box No.............

Lens No.	Power	Flat or curved	Form

TEST 2

Time allowed

Thirty minutes.

Lens set

Flat astigmatic set.

Instructions

You are required to record the identification number, power and axis direction, *in the form in which the lens has been made,* of any six sphero-cylindrical lenses selected from the accompanying box.

Record your results as follows.

Name. . . . . Group. . . . . Date. . . . .

Box No. . . . .

Lens No.	Sphere	Cylinder	Axis	Sph. + cyl.

You must complete the first four columns of the results table. The fifth column will be ignored by the examiner. It is provided for you to write down the second principal power of the lens if you use test spheres alone.

Note. – The engraved 180 meridians of the lens are marked on the front surface in each case.

TEST 3

Time allowed

Thirty minutes.

Lens set

Edged toric set.

Instructions

You are required to record the identification number, power, axis direction and sphere curve of any five edged toric lenses selected from the accompanying box.

APPENDIX 1

Record your results as follows.

Name............... Group............. Date.............
Box No.............

Lens No.	Sphere	Cylinder	Axis	Sph. curve

TEST 4

Time allowed

Thirty minutes.

Lens set

Marking and setting.

Instructions

You are required to lay-off each of the two pairs of lenses in the accompanying box according to the instructions given inside the lid. The lenses are not to be decentred. The prescriptions of the lenses have been written in the forms in which the lenses have been made, and you should be able to identify the lenses by inspection.

You should use ink or grease pencil. The cutting lines must be neat and accurate.

TEST 5

Time allowed

Thirty minutes.

Lens set

Edged toric set.

Instructions

You are required to record the identification number, power and axis direction of any five edged toric lenses selected from the

373

accompanying box. You must use only the lens measure in order to find the power. Record also the sphere curve of the lens.

Record your results as follows.

Name. . . . . Group. . . . . Date. . . . .
Box No. . . . .

Lens No.	Sphere	Cylinder	Axis	Sph. curve

Note. – You are advised to select minus lenses or low power lenses for this test.

TEST 6

Time allowed

Thirty minutes.

Lens set

Edged decentred lenses.

Instructions

You are required to record the identification number, power and axis direction, and the position of the optical centre in relation to the datum centre, of four edged decentred lenses selected from the accompanying box.

Record your results as follows.

Name. . . . . Group. . . . . Date. . . . .
Box No. . . . .

Lens No.	Sph.	Cylinder	Axis	Decentration from DC

TEST 7

Time allowed

Thirty minutes.

Lens set

Glazed frames SV.

Instructions

You are required to record the identification number and prescription of two pairs of glazed lenses by neutralization. The position of the optical centre in relation to the datum centre should be given.

Record your results as follows.

Name................ Group............ Date............
Box No..............

Frame No.	Sph.	Cyl.	Axis	Decentration
	R.			
	L.			

TEST 8

Time allowed

Twenty minutes.

Lens set

Glazed frames SV.

Instructions

You are required to record the identification number and prescription of two pairs of glazed lenses by means of the focimeter. The position of the optical centre in relation to the datum centre should be given.

Record your results as follows.

Name. . . . .   Group. . . . .   Date. . . . .
Box No. . . . .

Frame No.	Sph.	Cyl.	Axis	Decentration
R.				
L.				

TEST 9

Time allowed

Thirty minutes.

Lens set

Marking and setting, bifocals.

Instructions

You are required to lay-off each of the two pairs of bifocal lenses in the accompanying box according to the instructions given inside the lid. The lenses can be identified, from the details given, by inspection.

You should use ink or grease pencil. The cutting lines must be neat and accurate.

TEST 10

Time allowed

Forty minutes.

Lens set

Bifocals in frames.

Instructions

You are required to record the identification number, prescription and segment details of two pairs of glazed bifocal lenses by neutralization.

Record your results as follows.

Name.............. Group............. Date............

Box No.............

Lens No.	Sph.	Cyl.	Axis	Add	Bifocal type	Seg. diam. or size	Seg. top position	Geom. inset	Bod. de(of OD from D(
R.									
L.									

TEST 11

Time allowed

Twenty minutes.

Lens set

Verification set and card.

Instructions

The spectacles in the accompanying box are assumed to have been supplied in accordance with the prescription and specification on the card bearing the same number. Examine and verify all details of the spectacles and record any errors or faults which you find in the spectacles.

Record your results as follows.

Name............... Group............. Date............

Rx No..............

Errors or faults in lenses:

Errors or faults in frame:

State here which of the above errors you could correct in the fitting room with the patient present.

TEST 12

Time allowed

Forty minutes.

Lens set

Bifocals in frames.

Instructions

You are required to record the identification number, prescription and segment details of two pairs of glazed bifocal lenses by means of the focimeter.

Record your results as follows.

Name.............. Group............ Date...........
Box No.............

Lens No.	Sph.	Cyl.	Axis	Add	Bifocal type	Seg. diam. or size	Seg. top position	Geom. inset	Bod. dec of OD from DC
R.									
L.									

Appendix 2

SCHEME OF ASSESSMENT

TEST 1

The student is required to record in exactly 30 minutes the identification number, prescription and form of ten spherical lenses from an assorted box. Before the test commences, please ensure that the students understand exactly what they are required to do and have drawn up a results sheet, as shown on their instruction forms.

Marks are to be allocated as follows:

Lens power correct ... 5
Lens form correct ... 2

This marking allows a maximum of 7 marks for each lens, with a maximum final total of 70.

Deduct marks as follows for incorrect answers:

Error in power limited to ± 0.25 D ... ... deduct 2
Error in power limited to ± 0.50 D ... ... deduct 3
Failure to put in sign or wrong sign ... ... deduct 5

Deduct up to a maximum of 5 marks from the final total for untidy or illegible presentation.

Example

Lens No.	Power	Flat or curved	Form
2.7	– 2.25	Curved	Periscopic

TEST 2

The student is required to record in exactly 30 minutes the identification number, prescription in the actual form in which the lens has been made, and axis direction of six sphero-cylindrical lenses selected from the set of ten lenses. Before the test commences, please ensure that the students understand exactly what they are required to do and have drawn up a results sheet as shown on their instruction forms.

Marks are to be allocated as follows:

Sphere power correct	...	3
Cylinder power correct	...	3
Axis correct	...	3

This marking allows a maximum of 9 marks for each lens, with a maximum final total of 54.

Deduct marks as follows for incorrect answers:

Error in sph. or cyl. power limited to ± 0.25 D ...	deduct	1
Error in sph. or cyl. power limited to ± 0.50 D ...	deduct	2
Error in axis limited to ± 5°	deduct	1
Error in axis limited to ± 10°	deduct	2

If sign is missing or incorrect, wrong form is recorded or axis is 90° off, deduct all marks. Ignore fifth column of student's results table.

Deduct up to a maximum of 5 marks from the final total for untidy or illegible presentation.

TEST 3

The student is required to record in exactly 30 minutes the identification number, prescription and sphere curve of five edged toric lenses, using a neutralizing set and a lens measure. Before the test commences, please ensure that the students understand exactly what they are required to do and have drawn up a results sheet as shown on their instruction forms.

Marks are to be allocated as follows:

Sphere power correct	...	3
Cylinder power correct	...	3
Axis correct	...	3
Sphere curve correct	...	2

This marking allows a maximum of 11 marks for each lens, with a maximum final total of 55.

Deduct marks as follows for incorrect answers:

Error in sph. or cyl. power limited to ± 0.25 D ...	deduct 1
Error in sph. or cyl. power limited to ± 0.50 D ...	deduct 2
Error in axis limited to ± 5°	deduct 1
Error in axis limited to ± 10°	deduct 2
Error in sphere curve limited to ± 0.25 D ...	deduct 1

If sign is missing or incorrect or axis is 90° off, deduct all marks. Deduct up to a maximum of 5 marks from the final total for untidy or illegible presentation.

TEST 4

The student is required to lay-off two pairs of lenses for glazing according to the instructions given inside the lid of the box. He should be able to identify the lenses by inspection. Exactly 30 minutes should be allowed. Before the test commences, please ensure that the students understand exactly what they are required to do.

Marks should be allocated as follows.

Correct lens marked ...	1
Axis and optical centre correct ...	2
Horizontal cutting line correct ...	2
Vertical cutting line correct ...	2
Arrowhead on nasal side ...	1
R. or L. in temporal corner ...	1

This marking allows a maximum of 9 marks for each lens, with a maximum final total of 36.

Deduct marks as follows for incorrect answers:

Axis up to 5° off	deduct 1
Cutting lines not straight	deduct 2
	(1 for each lens)
Cutting lines not passing through OC	deduct 2

No marks are to be allocated for the following faults:

Wrong lens marked.
Wrong surface marked (laying off on front surface only).
Axis over 5° off.

TEST 5

The student is required to record in exactly 30 minutes the identification number, prescription and sphere curve of five edged toric lenses, using only a lens measure. Before the test commences, please ensure that the students understand exactly what they are required to do and have drawn up a results sheet as shown on their instruction forms.

Marks are to be allocated as follows:

Sphere power correct	... 3
Cylinder power correct	... 3
Axis correct	... 3
Sphere curve correct	... 2

This marking allows a maximum of 11 marks for each lens, with a maximum final total of 55.

Deduct marks as follows for incorrect answers:

Error in sphere power limited to ± 0.25 D	... deduct 0
Error in cylinder power limited to ± 0.25 D	... deduct 1
Error in sph. or cyl. power limited to ± 0.50 D ...	deduct 2
Error in axis limited to ± 5°	... ... deduct 1
Error in axis limited to ± 10°	... ... deduct 2
Error in sphere curve limited to ± 0.25 D	... deduct 1

If sign is missing or incorrect, wrong form is recorded or axis is 90° off, deduct all marks.

Deduct up to a maximum of 5 marks from the final total for untidy or illegible presentation.

TEST 6

The student is required to record in exactly 30 minutes the identification number, power and axis direction, and the position of the optical centre in relation to the datum centre, of four edged decentred lenses. Before the test commences, please ensure that the students understand exactly what they are required to do and have drawn up a results sheet as shown on their instruction forms.

Marks are to be allocated as follows:

Sphere power correct	... 3
Cylinder power correct	... 3
Axis correct	... 3
Decentration correct	... 4

This marking allows a maximum of 13 marks for each lens, with a maximum final total of 52.

Deduct marks as follows for incorrect answers:

Error in sph. or cyl. power limited to ± 0.25 D . . .	deduct 1
Error in sph. or cyl. power limited to ± 0.50 D . . .	deduct 2
Error in axis limited to ± 5°	deduct 1
Error in axis limited to ± 10°	deduct 2
Error in vertical decentration limited to 1 mm . . .	deduct 1
Error in vertical decentration limited to 2 mm . . .	deduct 2
Error in horizontal decentration limited to 1 mm	deduct 1
Error in horizontal decentration limited to 2 mm	deduct 2

If sign is missing or incorrect or axis is 90° off, deduct all marks.

Deduct up to a maximum of 5 marks from the final total for untidy or illegible presentation.

TEST 7

The student is required to record in exactly 30 minutes the identification number, prescription and position of the optical centre of two pairs of glazed lenses by means of neutralization. Before the test commences, please ensure that the students understand exactly what they are required to do and have drawn up a results sheet as shown on their instruction forms.

Marks are to be allocated as follows:

Sphere power correct	. . .	3
Cylinder power correct	. . .	3
Axis correct	. . .	3
Decentration correct	. .	3

This marking allows a maximum of 12 marks for each lens (24 marks per pair), with a maximum final total of 48.

Deduct marks as follows for incorrect answers:

Error in sph. or cyl. power limited to ± 0.25 D . . .	deduct 1
Error in sph. or cyl. power limited to ± 0.50 D . . .	deduct 2
Error in axis limited to ± 5°	deduct 1
Error in axis limited to ± 10°	deduct 2
Error in decentration limited to 1 mm	deduct 1
Error in decentration limited to 2 mm	deduct 2

If sign is missing or incorrect, axis is 90° off or wrong eye prescription is recorded, deduct all marks.

Deduct up to a maximum of 5 marks from the final total for untidy or illegible presentation.

TEST 8

The student is required to record in exactly 30 minutes the identification number, prescription and position of the optical centre of two pairs of glazed lenses by means of the focimeter. Before the test commences, please ensure that the students understand exactly what they are required to do and have drawn up a results sheet as shown on their instruction forms.

Marks are to be allocated as follows:

Sphere power correct ...	2
Cylinder power correct ...	2
Axis correct ...	3
Decentration correct ...	3

This marking allows a maximum of 10 marks for each lens (20 marks per pair), with a maximum final total of 40.

Deduct marks as follows for incorrect answers:

Error in sph. or cyl. power limited to ± 0.25 D ...	deduct 1
Error in axis limited to ± 5°	deduct 1
Error in axis limited to ± 10°	deduct 2
Error in decentration limited to 1 mm	deduct 1
Error in decentration limited to 2 mm	deduct 2

If sign is missing or incorrect, axis is 90° off or wrong eye prescription is recorded, deduct all marks.

Deduct up to a maximum of 5 marks from the final total for untidy or illegible presentation.

TEST 9

The student is required to lay-off two pairs of bifocal lenses for glazing in exactly 30 minutes. The instructions for the lenses are given in the box lids. The student should be able to identify the lenses by inspection. Before the test commences, please ensure that the students understand exactly what they are required to do.

Marks should be allocated as follows:

Correct lens marked ...	1
Axis and optical centre correct ...	2

Horizontal cutting line correct (seg. top position)	...	2
Vertical cutting line correct (geom. inset)	...	2
Arrowhead on nasal side	...	1
R. or L. in temporal corner	...	1
Segments match from cutting lines (when R. lens matched with L. lens)	...	1

This marking allows a maximum of 10 marks for each lens, with a final maximum total of 40.

Deduct marks as follows for incorrect answers:

Error in axis limited to ± 5° ...	deduct 1 for each lens
Error in seg. top position limited to 0.5 mm	deduct 1 for each lens
Error in geom. inset limited to 1 mm	deduct 1 for each lens

If the segments do not match when held front to front with cutting lines in alignment, deduct 2 marks from the pair (1 mark for each lens).

No marks are to be allocated for the following faults:

Wrong lens marked.
Wrong surface marked.

TEST 10

The student is required to record in exactly 30 minutes the identification number, prescription, segment type and details of two pairs of glazed bifocal lenses. Before the test commences, please ensure that the students understand exactly what they have to do and have drawn up a results sheet as shown on their instruction forms.

Marks are to be allocated as follows:

Sphere power correct	... 2	Bifocal type correct	... 1
Cylinder power correct	... 2	Seg. diam. or size correct	... 1
Axis correct	... 2	Seg. top position correct	... 2
Reading Add correct	... 2	Geom. inset correct	... 2
Bod. dec. of dist. OC correct	... 1		

This marking allows a maximum of 15 marks for each lens (30 marks per pair), with a maximum final total of 60.

SCHEME OF ASSESSMENT

Deduct marks as follows for incorrect answers:

Error in sph., cyl. or Add limited to ± 0.25 D	...	deduct 1 for each error
Error in axis limited to ± 5°	... ...	deduct 1
Error in seg. top position limited to 0.5 mm	...	deduct 1
Error in geom. inset limited to 1 mm	... ...	deduct 1

If sign is missing or incorrect, axis is 90° off or wrong eye prescription is recorded, deduct all marks.

Deduct up to a maximum of 5 marks from the final total for untidy or illegible presentation.

TEST 11

The student is required to assume that the spectacles which he has been given have been made in accordance with the specification on the accompanying card. He is required to examine and verify all details of the spectacles and record any errors or faults which he finds. He should also state which errors he could correct in the fitting room, using the usual equipment which he would find in the fitting room. The time allowed is 20 minutes.

Before the test commences, please ensure that the students understand exactly what they are required to do and have drawn up a results sheet as shown on their instruction forms.

Marks should be allocated as indicated on the answer sheets for this experiment and expressed as a percentage.

Deduct up to a maximum of 10 per cent from the final total for untidy or illegible presentation.

TEST 12

The student is required to record in exactly 40 minutes the identification number, prescription, segment type and details of two pairs of glazed bifocal lenses by means of the focimeter. Before the test commences, please ensure that the students understand exactly what they have to do and have drawn up a results sheet as shown on their instruction forms.

Marks are to be allocated as follows:

Sphere power correct	... 2	Bifocal type correct	... 1
Cylinder power correct	... 2	Seg. diam. or size correct	... 1
Axis correct	... 2	Seg. top position correct	... 2
Reading Add correct	... 2	Geom. inset correct	... 2
Bod. dec. of dist. OC correct	... 1		

This marking allows a maximum of 15 marks for each lens (30 marks per pair), with a maximum final total of 60.

Deduct marks as follows for incorrect answers:

Error in sph., cyl. or Add limited to $\pm$ 0.25 D ... deduct 1 for each error

Error in axis limited to $\pm$ 5° ... ... deduct 1

Error in seg. top position limited to 0.5 mm ... deduct 1

Error in geom. inset limited to 1 mm ... ... deduct 1

If sign is missing or incorrect, axis is 90° off or wrong eye prescription is recorded, deduct all marks.

Deduct up to a maximum of 5 marks from the final total for untidy or illegible presentation.

Appendix 3

EXAMPLES OF COMPUTER PROGRAMS AND OUTPUT, AND PROGRAMS FOR PROGRAMMABLE CALCULATORS

To determine the front central optic radius (see Experiment 96)

Figure A3.1. Flow diagram and program for Texas SR52 calculator

TEXAS INSTRUMENTS
SR 52 program to find r_1, given F'_v, t, r_2.

Step	Key	Code	Step	Key	Code
000	2nd LBL	46	026	0	00
001	A	11	027	4	04
002	STO	42	028	$+/-$	94
003	0	00	029	$+$	85
004	2	02	030	RCL	43
005	HLT	81	031	0	00
006	2nd LBL	46	032	2	02
007	C	13	033	$=$	95
008	STO	42	034	2nd $\frac{1}{x}$	20
009	0	00	035	EE	52
010	3	03	036	3	03
011	HLT	81	037	$+$	85
012	2nd LBL	46	038	(	53
013	D	14	039	RCL	43
014	STO	42	040	0	00
015	0	00	041	3	03
016	4	04	042	$\div$	55
017	HLT	81	043	1	01
018	2nd LBL	46	044		93
019	B	12	045	4	04
020	4	04	046	9	09
021	9	09	047	)	54
022	0	00	048	$=$	95
023	$+/-$	94	049	$\times$	65
024	$\div$	55	050		93
025	RCL	43	051	4	04
			052	9	09
			053	$=$	95
			054	HLT	81

(continued on page 368)

388

Figure A3.1 (Continued)

Step 1.

Enter F'_v	Press A	Display F'_v
Enter $t$mm	Press C	Display t
Enter $r_2$mm	Press D	Display r^2

Step 2.

Calculate r_1 Press B   Display r_1
  Equation from which program is derived is:

$$r_1 = (n-1)\left(\frac{1000}{F'_v - F_2} + \frac{t}{n}\right)$$

where n is refractive index.
r_1, radius of front CL surface in mm.
F'_v, back vertex power in dioptres.
t = thickness of lens in mm and

$$F_2 = \frac{(1-n)1000}{r_2}$$

where r_2 is radius of back CL surface.

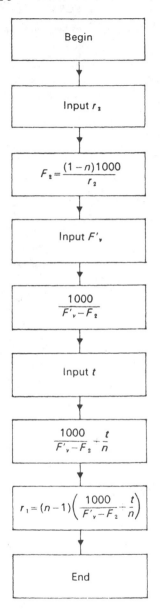

Figure A3.2. Flow diagram and program for HP67 calculator

HP 67 program to determine front surface radius of a contact lens.
The flowchart in Figure 10 shows the sequence of operation for this program.

STEP No	PROGRAM INSTRUCTION	EXPLANATION
001	f LBL A	Starting address
002	1	
003	·	
004	4	generate the refractive index, n, 1·49
005	9	
006	STO 0	store ref. index in Reg. 0
007	1	generate 1
008	−	evaluate $n-1$
009	RCL 0	recall n from Reg. 0
010	÷	evaluate $(n-1)/n$
011	STO 1	store $(n-1)/n$ in Reg 1
012	RCL 0	recall n from Reg. 0
013	×	evaluate $(n-1)$
014	EEX	
015	3	generate 1000 (10^3)
016	×	evaluate 1000 $(n-1)$
017	STO 3	store 1000 $(n-1)$ in Reg. 3
018	R/S	stop to enter F'_v
019	R/S	stop to enter r_s
020	CHS	change the sign of r_s
021	STO ÷ 3	evaluate F_s in Reg. 3
022	CLX	clear the X Reg.
023	RCL 3	recall F_s from Reg. 3
024	−	evaluate $F'_v - F_s$
025	÷	evaluate $r_1 n$
026	R/S	stop to enter t
027	RCL 1	recall $(n-1)/n$ from Reg. 1
028	×	evaluate $t(n-1)/n$
029	+	evaluate r_1
030	h RTN	end program execution

Figure A3.3. Program listing in BASIC, and resultant output

```
100 PRINT"THIS PROGRAM CALCULATES.THE FRONT"
110 PRINT"CENTRAL OPTIC RADIUS GIVEN THE"
120 PRINT"BACK CENTRAL OPTIC RADIUS R2"
130 PRINT"BACK VERTEX POWER,AND CENTRAL"
140 PRINT"THICKNESS T MM,REF.INDEX ASSUMED"
150 PRINT"TO BE 1.49"
160 PRINT
170 PRINT"TYPE BACK CENTRAL OPIC RADIUS R2"
180 PRINT
190 INPUT R2
200 PRINT
210 PRINT"TYPE BACK VERTEX POWER"
220 PRINT
230 INPUT V
240 PRINT
250 PRINT"TYPE CENTRAL THICKNESS,MM"
260 PRINT
270 .INPUT T
280 PRINT
290 LET N=1.49
300 LET F2=(1-N)*1000/R2
310 LET R1=(N-1)*((1000/(V-F2))+T/N)
320 LET R=INT(100*R1+0.5)/100
330 PRINT
340 PRINT"FRONT CENTRAL OPTIC RADIUS IS";R"MM"
350 END


RUN
THIS PROGRAM CALCULATES THE FRONT
CENTRAL OPTIC RADIUS GIVEN THE
BACK CENTRAL OPTIC RADIUS R2
BACK VERTEX POWER,AND CENTRAL
THICKNESS T MM,REF.INDEX ASSUMED
TO BE 1.49

TYPE BACK CENTRAL OPIC RADIUS R2

? 8

TYPE BACK VERTEX POWER

? 0
```

```
TYPE CENTRAL THICKNESS,MM

? 0.6


FRONT CENTRAL OPTIC RADIUS IS 8.2 MM


RUN 160-

TYPE BACK CENTRAL OPIC RADIUS R2

? 8

TYPE BACK VERTEX POWER

? 1.52

TYPE CENTRAL THICKNESS,MM

? 0.6


FRONT CENTRAL OPTIC RADIUS IS 8 MM


RUN 160

TYPE BACK CENTRAL OPIC RADIUS R2

? 7.83

TYPE BACK VERTEX POWER

? -4.25


TYPE CENTRAL THICKNESS,MM

? 0.15


FRONT CENTRAL OPTIC RADIUS IS 8.45 MM
```

Program listing in BASIC to determine horizontal and vertical decentrations for given horizontal and vertical prisms, and resultant output

```
100   PRINT "TYPE R FOR RE L FOR LE"
110   INPUT A$
120   PRINT "ENTER SPH"
130   INPUT S
140   PRINT "ENTER CYL"
150   INPUT C
160   PRINT "ENTER AXIS"
170   INPUT B
180   LET A=B*3.14159/180
190   PRINT "ENTER HOR PRISM CHANGE SIGN IF BASE IN"
200   INPUT H
210   PRINT "ENTER VERT PRISM CHANGE SIGN IF BASE DOWN"
220   INPUT V
230   IF A$="R" THEN 250
240   LET A=3.14159-A
250   LET X=(H*S+(H*C*COS(A)^2)-V*C*SIN(A)*COS(A))/(S*(S+C))
260   LET Y=(V*S+(V*C*SIN(A)^2)-H*C*SIN(A)*COS(A))/(S*(S+C))
270   LET X1=INT(X*100+.5)/100
280   LET Y1=INT(Y*100+.5)/100
290 PRINT X1;" CM IS HOR DEC, IN IF NEGATIVE"
300 PRINT Y1;" CM IS VERT DEC, DOWN IF NEGATIVE"
310   END


TYPE R FOR RE L FOR LE
!R
ENTER SPH
!-2.25
ENTER CYL
!2.75
ENTER AXIS
!60
ENTER HOR PRISM CHANGE SIGN IF BASE IN
!-4
ENTER VERT PRISM CHANGE SIGN IF BASE DOWN
!3
-2.37 CM IS HOR DEC, IN IF NEGATIVE
-3.72 CM IS VERT DEC, DOWN IF NEGATIVE

TYPE R FOR RE L FOR LE
!L
ENTER SPH
!-2.25
ENTER CYL
!2.75
ENTER AXIS
!120
ENTER HOR PRISM CHANGE SIGN IF BASE IN
!-4
ENTER VERT PRISM CHANGE SIGN IF BASE DOWN
!3
-2.37 CM IS HOR DEC, IN IF NEGATIVE
-3.72 CM IS VERT DEC, DOWN IF NEGATIVE
```

Program listing in BASIC to give a table of edge thickness difference of a prism, and resultant output (see Experiment 37)

```
10    PRINT "                                          TABLE"
20    PRINT "OF EDGE THICKNESS DIFFERENCE"
30    PRINT "OF A PRISM"
40    PRINT
50    PRINT "REFRACTIVE INDEX"
60    INPUT N
65    PRINT
70    PRINT "Prism"TAB(35), "Diameter (mm.)"
75    PRINT "Dioptres                    50                        52";
80    PRINT "                54              56              58"
85    PRINT
90    FOR P=7 TO 10 STEP .25
100   PRINT P,
110   LET T=8
120   FOR D=50 TO 58 STEP 2
130   LET G=D*P/100/((N*SQR(1+(P/100)^2))-1)
140   LET G1=INT(G*100+.5)/100
150   PRINT TAB(T);G1;
160   LET T=T+8
170   NEXT D
180   PRINT
190   NEXT P
200   END
```

TABLE
OF EDGE THICKNESS DIFFERENCE
OF A PRISM

REFRACTIVE INDEX
?1.523

Prism Dioptres	Diameter (mm.)				
	50	52	54	56	58
7	6.64	6.91	7.18	7.44	7.71
7.25	6.88	7.15	7.43	7.7	7.98
7.5	7.11	7.4	7.68	7.97	8.25
7.75	7.35	7.64	7.93	8.23	8.52
8	7.58	7.88	8.18	8.49	8.79
8.25	7.81	8.12	8.43	8.75	9.06
8.5	8.04	8.36	8.69	9.01	9.33
8.75	8.27	8.6	8.94	9.27	9.6
9	8.5	8.84	9.18	9.52	9.86
9.25	8.73	9.08	9.43	9.78	10.13
9.5	8.96	9.32	9.68	10.04	10.4
9.75	9.19	9.56	9.93	10.3	10.67
10	9.42	9.8	10.18	10.55	10.93

The authors wish to thank the Editor of *The Optician* for permission to reproduce items (A1) and (A2) from their article in *The Optician*, No. 4523, Vol. 175: 'Using programmable calculators in the practice and workshop'.

INDEX